RECOVERING FROM THE GAME

RECOVERING FROM THE GAME

RICHARD BEAL

This book is dedicated to all the people who have gone through the Game and are recovering, receiving a second chance at a first-class life.

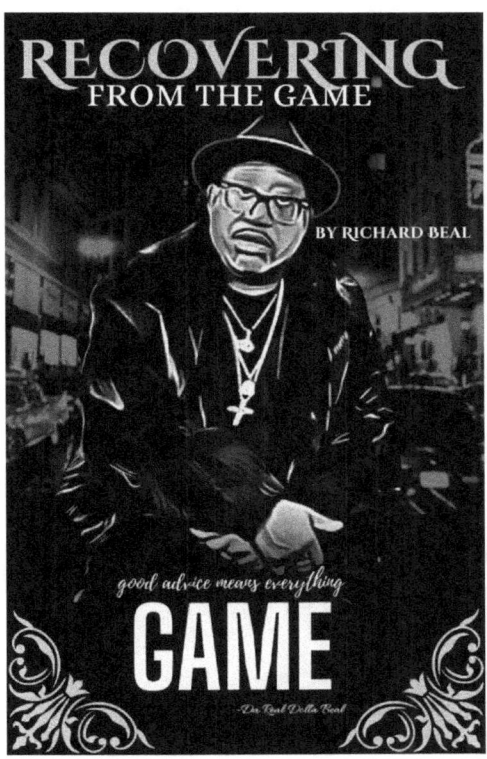

CONTENTS

Foreword

I first met Richard Beal in 1997. I remember him walking into the room with a big smile on his face and the swagger that I recognized immediately as that of somebody who was familiar with "the game." He had a contagious twinkle in his eyes and the gift of gab, but instead of talking drag, he was talking recovery. He was clearly on a mission for his recovery the same way he was on a mission to get his money. I was immediately struck and impressed with this brother, and he was a reminder that recovery doesn't make you a new person, it makes you a better version of your old self. Over the years I've seen many players and hustlers come into the rooms of recovery and apply their old skill set into something positive. Richard Beal, a.k.a. the Ambassador for Recovery, is a testament to that. This book illustrates that there's a whole bunch of us out there who found a way out of the darkness of the game and into the light of recovery. Much love to you, Richard "Dollar Bill" Beal.

-- Roland "RoDog" Williams

Introduction

For over 20 years I dreamed of writing this book, and now that dream has finally become a reality. *Recovering From The Game* is more than just a collection of stories; it's a testament to the power of transformation and the resilience of the human spirit. This journey would not have been possible without the help and support of many incredible individuals. I owe a heartfelt thank you to my co-writer, Mark Grey, and to everyone who was brave enough to share their stories and experiences in these pages.

A special "Thank You" to Randy Shaw, Founder of Tenderloin Housing Clinic, who inspired me as a trailblazer, author, and activist, always standing up for what he believes in no matter what.

This book is for anyone who has ever felt trapped in the game—once a life defined by hustling, addiction, and struggle. Today, GAME stands for *Good Advice Means Everything*. It's a reflection of how far we've come and a guide to how far we can go. This book is my way of saying to all the pimps, players, hustlers, and gangsters: *we do recover.* As the saying goes, "lost dreams awaken, and new possibilities arise."

My personal journey began when I entered recovery at 29 years old. Up until that point, I had never held a legitimate job. Recovery gave me not just a new start, but a second chance at a first-class life. I'm forever grateful to the God of my understanding for the opportunity to rewrite my story.

If there's one thing I hope readers take away from this book, it's that addiction does not have to define you. You don't have to numb your pain with drugs, alcohol, food, gambling, sex, or material possessions. There is a way out, and there is a life beyond the horrors of addiction. Recovery is possible for anyone willing to take the steps, and *Recovering From The Game* is here to show you that change is not just achievable—it's inevitable when you commit to it.

This book is for you, for all of us. Because together, we recover.

CHAPTER 1

Richard Beal a.k.a. "Dollar Bill"

M an, I have something that I want to talk about here. You know, I was infatuated with the game and everything that went along with it from seein' my father and all the other men I grew up watching as a kid. I went from hustling in Richmond to hustling in Oakland, and then finally making my way out here to San Francisco in the early '80s. In the '80s I came out to San Francisco just coppin' dope, and I never knew much about recovery. I heard people talking about going to church, and I knew about Glide Church specifically, because Glide was goin' strong back then as well. But when I came out to the Tenderloin, I came out here to cop me some dope. I ended up coming out here and I eventually became homeless, living on the street for a number of years.

I would get a hotel room, and hustle out of my hotel room. I would also get a general assistance check, and the GA checks would always come to the check cashing place at twelve o'clock midnight. So, at twelve o'clock midnight, the dope dealers would be at the check cashing place with a line of rocks right outside the check cashing spot, and I'm talkin' a *line* of crack rocks. There would be a line of people at the check cashing place waiting to get their GA checks. At 12:01AM, the check cashing place would issue out their checks, and the dope dealers would be sellin' dope before people even got their check. Dealers were doing stuff on consignment because the money was just a few feet away. When people got their check, they'd just buy their dope right outside the door of the check cashing spot. Man, it was so bad that people would spend their entire check before it got daylight again. They'd be busted broke in just a few hours. This happened to me a few times those days when I would go on a binge and was totally out of control. I just smoked up all my money that night. All of us who did that would have to wait another two weeks, or another thirty days, for our next check, and do it all over again.

A lot of people who saw me living like this told me that I needed to go to Glide. They told me that I needed to go to the Men in Motion group. "Hey man, they got Positive Directions goin' on. Hey man, you need to go to the Salvation Army. They'll take anybody man, they got a work program out there. You need to go St. Anthony's. Hey man, you need to get some rest, you look tore up, you've been up for two or three days." I would listen, and on occasion I'd check out some of these places. I'd get my detox on, stay a night or two, get some rest like people said I should. I remember people talking about all the services that were going on in San Francisco, and Glide offered the most. They had a lot of support groups that friends of mine had gotten clean with, like Facts on Crack, Men in Motion, The Gathering with Positive Directions. I also heard about The Smith House and programs on Treasure Island, and then there was this 30-day program group called Tom Smith that was set up in General Hospital. I'd heard about all of these places and programs where you could get clean, so when I finally made a decision to get clean, I went to St. Anthony's on July 18, 1995, and the last time I used was the 17th. The 18th was my first day clean. July 18, 1995.

My first memory getting introduced to the life was when I was nine years old. But a whole lot happened to me, my five brothers, and four sisters before then. We got disconnected when I was six months old, when my father went to the penitentiary and my mother went back to Mississippi, leaving us in a shelter until our great-aunt adopted us. My father was sentenced to five-to-life with nineteen counts of armed robbery.

When my mother went back to Mississippi, my father said that was all fine and good, but his boys were to stay out in California with my aunt and my mother. At the time I had three older brothers. I had William, one year older than me; Larry, two years older than me; and Anthony, three years older than me. In 1965, my mother was only twenty years old, with four kids. Twenty years old, four kids, she'd had my oldest brother at seventeen. She was just a baby herself, and her old man went to prison. So, she went back to her mother. For a long time I had a resentment toward my mother for leaving me. How can you leave your six-month-old baby? Then in my recovery I did an examination of my life. I was able to look at my mother's situation in a different light after some time. I started seeing my mother again. I would go out to Mississippi and visit her. Me and my mother had a beautiful relationship when she passed away.

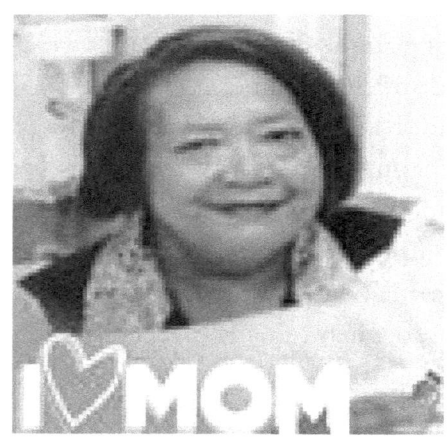

My mother, Ella Mae

While my mother was in Mississippi, she met a man named Earnest McDonald, and she had three more kids. So that's how I got my three sisters. My father got out of the penitentiary in 1970 after around five years, because his crime partner who snitched on him causing him to get sentenced got caught up in a bunch of lies. My father got out and had my oldest sister, Melodie, in December 1970 with his new girl, Phillis Beckman. I still have a great relationship with Phillis and my stepsister Susie to this day. So, me and my three older brothers have the same mother and father, my two younger brothers have the same father, my oldest sister has the same father, and my younger three sisters have the same mother as me.

I grew up in California. I was born in Martinez, CA, and I grew up in Richmond.

When my father went to the penitentiary and my mom returned to Mississippi, my grandmother and auntie raised me and my brothers. First we actually went to a shelter for about a year because my grandmother had gotten sick. Before the system would let my aunt adopt us, they made her go through some kind of trial period, and while this was all happening me and my brothers were put into a shelter. To this day I re-

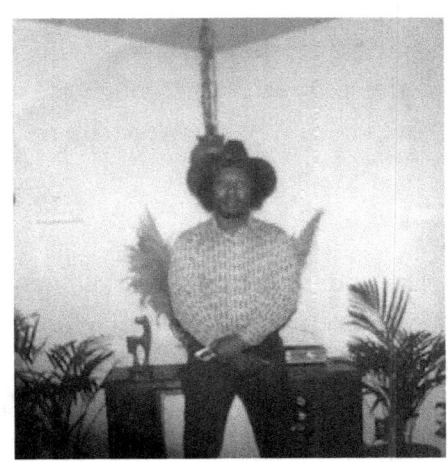

My father, Wild Willie Beal, around 1970

member that all we had to eat every morning at the shelter was powdered milk, powdered eggs, and Cheerios cereal. I hate Cheerios! To this day, I could be staying at somebody's house and they could have Honey Nut Cheerios, frosted Cheerios, they could have all kinds of fruity Cheerios, multigrain Cheerios, but I do not eat Cheerios! I say that as an example of how all those things that happened to me when I was little had a ripple effect on my whole life. Being abandoned, feeling like I was rejected by my mother. Having that resentment against my mother, having that separation from my father.

When my father got out of jail, I can remember him driving up in a Cadillac with the fifth wheel in the back. He had three young women in the backseat, and he was pimpin'. They called him "Wild Willie Bill" because he used to be a boxer in prison. Then he got out and started doing his thing. He was always in the game. That's all he ever knew. And all I knew my father to do was smoke weed. I never saw him drunk. I never saw him smoke cigarettes. I never saw him out of control in any way as far as any drugs or anything. My father could never figure out why all of his sons ended up becoming dope fiends. He couldn't figure out why we got caught up so bad, but at nine years old I'd started stealing the doobies out of his ashtray. He was selling weed, and when he would throw away the seeds we'd sift through the seeds and make joints out of what we could find. We'd try to pick up his scraps like some kids do.

Then our father started hooking up us boys with weed so we could sell it. At twelve years old I was selling fifty cent joints, five-dollar matchboxes, and three finger lids. And let me tell you, me and my brothers were running stuff. We were always in school together since we were just one year apart. If you had a problem with me—if you ran off with my money or you didn't pay me for something or you disrespected me—my first thing I would always do was punch you in the mouth. If I couldn't whoop you, I'd get my brothers and all of us would. This is how we lived for a very long time.

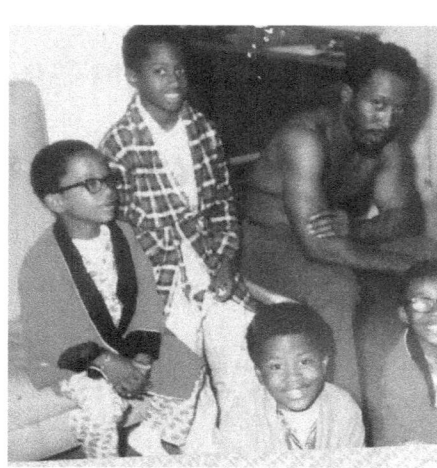

(clockwise from left) Me, Larry, Pops, Anthony, William

When we got into high school people found out that Willie Beal was our father, and he was the man in Richmond. I got kicked out of every high school I went to as a result of his reputation. I went to Harry Ells High School in Richmond, and I got kicked out of there for gang bangin' and fighting. I went to John F Kennedy, and I got kicked out of there for gang bangin' and fighting. I went to Richmond High, and I got kicked out of there for gang bangin' and fighting as well. I graduated from Richmond

High Adult School at night, because they said if they saw me in the day-time, they would call the police. My brothers went through the same thing I did. Two of my brothers ended up going to a continuation school in Richmond called Samuel Gompers. You see, my brothers and I and our friends were a gang, and everybody knew what would happen if we all went to the same school together.

I never had a job until I came into recovery. I just hustled. I admired the hustlers and pimps. Pimpin' wasn't my thing, but if a girl wanted to give me money, I'd take it. When they say *pimping ain't easy*, that's a true statement! It was too much drama with the women for me. One of my close partners went to jail because a girl he was pimpin' called the police. I was told by my father "don't trust these hoes." I liked hanging out with the pimps and the players because they had all the jewelry and all the money, and that's what was attractive to me. That pimp game wasn't my game, but I wanted what they had. What I really liked was the thrill of connin' somebody. I liked beating somebody with my mind, I would do the shortchange. I was good at sellin' junk, convincing someone that something is real when it isn't real. Fake jewelry, fake necklaces, fake watches, fake rings, you know, bricks in the box. I think we invented the bricks in the box—nobody in Richmond was doin' this until we came up with it. We'd get a new empty VCR box from a Best Buy, and we would wrap some bricks up, put them in the empty box so it felt like there was a brand-new VCR or laptop in the box. We'd go to a gas station and hook people up with these dummy boxes. "Hey man, I just hit Best Buy, look at all these brand-new VCRs I got. How many you want?" This was our thing. This was my biggest hustle back in the day.

When I wasn't doing that, I would set up a boost crew, and I used women for that. I'd have at least five or six women go into a store and just run in, take what they could, and run out. I think we invented that as well, and people are still doing that now. Go into Macy's with ten people, take as much shit as possible, and just get the hell out. There ain't enough security to chase ten women all at once.

My brother Anthony was the first one who started using hard drugs. At sixteen years old he was shootin' dope. My father put him out of the house after he found Anthony's needles. My brother Larry started committing burglaries, and he ended up going to the penitentiary. Then crack hit. My brother William got caught up in crack. First it was my brother William, and then it was me. All of us ended up on hard drugs. My drug of choice was crack, but I did everything else too. Every night, I wasn't above shootin' dope, snortin' dope, and doin' everything else. I was a garbage can.

That was my life until I came into recovery as a twenty-nine-year-old man. I did take breaks, going to detox. I went to my first meeting in 1983 at the Richmond Neighborhood House, a detox right there on 23rd Street and Richmond. I can remember it like it was yesterday. Everybody in there was older than me, they didn't look like me, they didn't sound like me. They were just washed up, didn't have no game. I was dishonest, closed-minded, and unwilling to change. I wasn't ready. My brother William had just gone through that same program. He had like eighteen months clean, and I saw him when he relapsed. He lost his car, he lost everything. So that taught me that if you relapse, it comes back worse than when you went in there.

After that detox I went through a number of transitions. I went from hustling in Richmond to hustling in Oakland and Berkeley, because at that time I was chasing the money and the dope. I would go from Oakland and Berkeley to San Francisco, to the Tenderloin. In 1986 I decided to join the Army. The Salvation Army. I went to the Salvation Army in 1986, man! And I did everything they told me not to do. I sold weed in the program, sold pills. I would go to the doctor, con him into giving me Tylenol with Codeine, and I would go back to the program and sell it. I would steal items at the Salvation Army loading docks. I would steal things from the Salvation Army auctions. When I got off work at the Salvation Army, I would go right around the corner and sell everything I'd stolen. I would go to all the little Chinese shops and sell them that slum jewelry that I had stolen. Of course the Salvation Army kicked me out, and that started a trend for me, man. From 1983 to 1995 I went in and out of detoxes and treatment centers, and I never was able to get thirty days clean. It took me twelve years to get thirty days. And I never was able to call any of that a relapse, because I had never really gotten clean.

I hit rock bottom in 1995 in the Tenderloin, and got myself to the St. Anthony's program at 55 Jones Street. It's closed now; the door doesn't even exist anymore. I went into detox on July 18, 1995. They had an NA meeting there, at 10:00, and on July 20 I went into the program. The last day I used was July 17, 1995. On the 17th, I lay in front of that door, and they let me in. I was too tore up to even do a full intake. They had me lay on a mat to let me sleep off the rest of the day. In the morning they checked on me, but they told me to keep sleeping because I was still too tore up for detox. On the 20th, this guy named Roy Washington was in the NA meeting and he said to me, "Are you ready? Are you ready to come into the program?" That's how I went into the St. Anthony's program.

Their recovery house, Seton Hall, was over at 165 Guerrero Street. I still have my graduation certificate from Seton Hall. That was a primary program for six months, and I did everything they told me to do. I worked in the dining room and then did treatment and went to groups in the evening. One day my brother William came by to visit me while I was at St. Anthony's, and he said, "Hey, I've got a handful of rocks, let's go!" But I said, "Hey man, I'm done." I knew then that if I could turn down my brother, I could turn down anybody. That was a turning point for me. I'll never forget it, man. It's been almost thirty years, and I remember it like it was yesterday.

They told me to go to ninety meetings in ninety days, but I think I went to a meeting every day for the first four or five years. Sometimes I was going to two or three meetings a day. I just really wanted to stay clean. I wanted to make my father proud, because he was still my hero even when he was still in the game. For a long time I wondered, *if my father can just smoke weed, why can't I do it?* I think that mindset kept me sick for a long time. Eventually I realized that I have the disease of addiction and my father didn't. I didn't know then that some people can drink all their lives, maybe just drink one drink a day, and never be an alcoholic. I never would be able to be like my father. I had to accept that.

I would read in the Big Book on page 449:

And acceptance is the answer to all my problems today. When I am disturbed, it is because I find some person, place, thing, or situation—some fact of my life—unacceptable to me, and I can find no serenity until I accept that person, place, thing, or situation as being exactly the way it is supposed to be at this moment. Nothing, absolutely nothing happens in God's world by mistake. Until I could accept my alcoholism, I could not stay sober; unless I accept life completely on life's terms, I cannot be happy. I need to concentrate not so much on what needs to be changed in the world as on what needs to be changed in me and in my attitudes.

I had to accept that I would never be able to just smoke weed. When I was able to accept that, my recovery went to another level. I listened when group facilitators said, "You're addicted to smokin'. You're addicted to that lifestyle. You were addicted to all that other stuff. Using is just a symptom of the disease of addiction." They said that people who stopped smoking had a better chance of staying clean, so I stopped smoking cigarettes in treatment. I completed the first three steps that were required for you to graduate the primary program. Since I was able to work through those first three steps and I was doing well, they allowed me to get a part-time job with St. Anthony's. I started saving my money, I built up my recovery network, I even had a roommate. Me and him are the only ones from that crew that are still clean today. We would all get passes to go outside to places like the zoo or to the farmer's market. Well, most of the other guys would lie about where they were going, and they would sneak off to see their girlfriends or hang out with their buddies. Me and my roommate, if we said we were going to the library, we went to the library. If we said we were going to the zoo, we went to the zoo. I wasn't going to get caught up in the stuff the other guys were getting into. Sure enough, one by one those other guys disappeared. Not me man, I was going to make it. I did my program to the best of my ability. Once I'd graduated from 165 Guerrero, Seton Hall, they let me into Covenant House.

Covenant House was one of the Victorian buildings over on Steiner Street, right across the street from Alamo Square, owned by St. Anthony's. It's a beautiful building still to this day. I graduated Covenant House, the secondary program, and I still have the certificate from that, too. But you know, some of those guys that were counselors in that program, I watched them relapse and die. Three of those counselors relapsed after many years of recovery. And every time somebody relapsed, it let me know that recovery is a one day at a time thing.

My first sponsor always told me that most people underestimate the disease of addiction and overestimate their recovery. They think that after a few years of sobriety, the same disease that used to whoop their ass back in the day, all of a sudden that same disease became a punk. So many people think they got the disease beat after a while. But my sponsor always used to tell me that this disease is cunning, baffling, powerful, and very patient. This disease will wait twenty, thirty years to get you. I listened to all of that.

When I first tried to get clean, people were doing that attack therapy stuff, but I never could get into that. I didn't get that "Sit down, shut the F up, if I want to hear from the disease, I'll talk to you" line. Because I always thought I had game, man. "What do you mean shut up? Man, my mouth got me money and got me through the world and now you are tellin' me to shut up?" In the beginning of my recovery, I would never have listened to all the suckers I was surrounded by. They had no game, man. I just couldn't get that. But people showed me unconditional love, and I learned that this whole thing is about one addict helping another. When I went to school years later, I was taught that that attack therapy approach was ineffective, that they had been tearing down people but didn't know how to build them back up. If you don't know how to build somebody back up, don't tear him down, man. So nobody even practices attack therapy anymore. Now it's about motivation, inspiring others, empathy, and meeting people where they are, and then bringing them up. It's about telling people: You *can* stop using, no matter what. It's the hugs and love that I received from the fellowship that really helped me in my recovery. I learned that it was about applying spiritual principles and learning how to be honest, open minded, and willing. I became committed to doing service and being in service in the city of San Francisco.

I was in a group called Men in Motion that met every Wednesday. We would circle, and we each had three minutes to talk about what we were going through and then got one minute feedback. We had that support group for years. It started in Glide Church, and eventually we moved over to 6th Street. Now that spot's an art center with a gallery, but the building is still there. We used to be on a radio show called *Soldiers in Recovery*. We met people like Danny Glover and Dr. Joe Marshall. I was entrenched in recovery for my first five years, either in treatment or transitional housing.

When I graduated the secondary program, I moved to 242 Turk Street, which is now the Salvation Army Kroc Center. At that time, it was Bridgeway Transitional Housing. You paid thirty percent of your income in rent, and you could stay there as long as you paid. Every week we were required to go to either AA or NA meetings that they had downstairs in the community room. They had a shelter downstairs too, where some of us would work. I lived at Bridgeway for three and a half years, just doing recovery every day. I had my men's support group. I was involved heavily in NA, and I even began facilitating groups. I would go to AA too, but NA was my thing. I was right in the belly of the beast, staying clean, going to meetings every day, doing what they told me to do, and I am grateful for Salvation Army.

Later I worked with Haight Ashbury Free Clinic, and that's when I got certified as a substance abuse counselor. I went to school at City College, completed the substance abuse program and the HIV program.

I went from being a counselor to a case manager, from a case manager to a program manager, and now I am director at Tenderloin Housing Clinic. I also ended up working in the San Francisco County Jail in San Bruno, California, for Center Point. I didn't really like working at the jail though, because seeing how people were treated in the system didn't sit well with me. I had made some of the same mistakes that those men on the inside made; I could have been one of those men. The only difference between me and those men sitting in prison is that they got caught and I didn't. Back in the day, my father would get me out of situations or someone else who knew someone in the system would get me out of another situation. When I worked inside the jail, I saw a lot of the same people that I used to run the streets with. I did a lot of the same crimes with some of those guys. They were in jail, and I was not. I didn't like working inside the criminal justice system all that much.

When I moved to Oakland, I got connected to NA's East Bay Fellowship, and within a year I was Chair of the East Bay Activities Committee. I was told that change isn't hard; it's the *resistance to change* that makes change hard. We started holding shows, barbeques, and picnics, and we started doing these big speaker jams. Each speaker would select a song for me to play while they walked up, then they'd speak after their song. We would dance with energy that was off the charts. We turned our recovery into theater, and we loved it.

I got married in early recovery. She had ninety days and I had three years, and it didn't work, man. She relapsed. Somebody called me one day and told me they saw my car in Lakeview. "What do you mean you saw my car in Lakeview?" They told me they knew it was my car because it had my NA bumper stickers on it. My wife had relapsed, and she stole my car, all my money, my jewelry, everything, man. I ended up getting an annulment after we'd been married for less than a year. I dusted myself off and went on with my recovery.

I met my second wife in recovery too. Gerri and I had already known each other in recovery because we had around the same clean time. Her clean date was July 9, 1995, and my clean date was July 18, 1995. She had gotten clean in Fresno, but she came back to San Francisco since she's from there. Gerri showed me that you don't have to go to treatment to get clean. She went to a 12-step meeting down in Fresno, then she stayed clean til the day she died. Nineteen years. She didn't go to treatment, she didn't do methadone, no outpatient, nothing. She did smoke cigarettes, and that ended up being the reason she had a heart attack. After we got married, we traveled all over the country together. We spoke at all the big meetings and speaker jams all over the country. We went to places like Dayton, Ohio; Pittsburgh, Pennsylvania; and Los Angeles, and we became this NA recovery power couple, popular on the speaker circuit. People would fly us in, put us up in a beautiful hotel room. We would speak at all the big conventions, like at Ocean City. I spoke at NCCNA in front of 3,000 people. That was our thing back then, man.

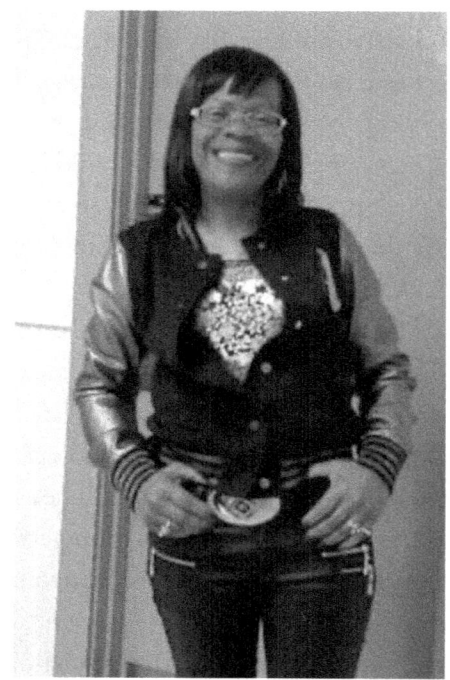

Gerri, always loved

I'll never forget December 14, 2014. We were living in Hayward, and Gerri wasn't feeling well. The week before that, the doctor had found a lump in her breast. I was going to take her to the hospital again because she still wasn't feeling well. As we were getting ready to leave, she just looked at me, she took a breath, and she went unconscious. I got her to the hospital, and they tried to bring her back, but they couldn't. Her time of death was 7:04am.

Losing Gerri was absolutely devastating for me. She was my soulmate. But her support group was really strong, and my support group was strong as well. People embraced me. The fellowship embraced me so much that I didn't have to do anything for her services. Everybody just joined in and took care of everything. Sponsors, sponsees, family and friends, everybody surrounded me and took care of me. People stopped by to make sure I was eating well. People talked to me to keep my spirits high and make sure I knew I wasn't alone. People picked me up to take me to meetings and make sure I was still connected to the program while getting through the loss of Gerri. So, eventually, I got through that.

Soon after Gerri passed away, my brother William was next. William had smoked a *lot* of crack. He passed away three days before his 46th birthday. We had gotten William into treatment at West Oakland Health Center, but he had a heart attack in the program. William went to the hospital after his heart attack, and then he never went back to the program. He would go into the Tenderloin in his wheelchair. Every time he got a little money, he would catch the BART from Oakland, make his way to the Tenderloin, and get himself some more crack. He died as a direct result of the disease of addiction.

William and I were just one year apart, same father, same mother. William was the one who had shown me that handful of rocks when I was in early recovery. For years I'd tried to show my brothers if I can do it, you can do it, but William and Anthony were never able to get clean. Anthony tried a geographic. He moved to Florida and to other places, and he would get clean for five or six months before he would relapse again. After Florida didn't work, I told Anthony to come back out and stay with me. Gerri had just died, so I had space for him even though he was still drinking and using. I had a three-bedroom apartment; he stayed in one room, I had one room, and I used my third room as an office. But when I went into Anthony's room on March 1, 2017, to check on him, I found him with his eyes open and foam coming out of both sides of his mouth. He'd had a diabetic seizure from drinking and using drugs. He was gone.

LaTonya, the beautiful woman who is my wife today, was a caregiver when I met her. I called her up when Anthony died, and she came over and cleaned up Anthony's face and his body. I called the police, who came and saw that he had overdosed. They didn't even call the medical examiner. They just dismissed the body directly over to me. To them it was just another dope fiend overdose. I called the funeral home so they would come over and pick him up. There were maybe ten people at Anthony's funeral. He was disconnected from everybody; he was just an addict dope fiend. It was sad, man. And you know, I still have both my brothers' ashes at my house right now. I offered William's ashes to his son Marcus, but he said he didn't want them.

LaTonya and I got married in 2017 on my birthday, so she was my birthday present. We went to Hawaii. I flew her mother and daughter out to Hawaii, and then my sponsor came to be my best man. We got married on the beach of Waikiki. I got an Airbnb for two weeks and let everyone stay in the Airbnb while LaTonya and I went on a cruise together. It was beautiful. We're still married today, man, and every year we get to celebrate our marriage on my birthday. She's not in recovery. She's a normie. But we have a beautiful, healthy relationship. LaTonya will tell her story later on in this book.

So, yeah man, in all that time I have been trying to work with people who are caught in the game selling drugs and doing some of the other things that I did. I still know some of the guys who were out there when I was out there hustling in Richmond and Oakland and San Francisco, like Candyman and Fillmore Slim. I used to hang out with the pimps and the players in Fillmore. People would say stuff like, "Hey Little Bill, check this out. There's only one requirement when it comes to pimpin'." I'd say, "What you talkin' about?" and they would say, "You gotta have a ho." I didn't care, because I was a hustler, and pimping was never my thing. They would say, "The game is to be sold and not told." But if they had told me what the game was, I never would have done it. If they had told me it was going to lead me to being homeless and tore up and disconnected from my family and my friends, all the things that

I went through and put other people through, I never would have done any of it.

When I didn't have a place to go, my father, God rest his soul, would always open his door and let me come back in. He put me out again sometimes, but he was always there for me. I can remember when my father told me he had cancer. He went into the hospital in July of 1999, and in September he was dead. He walked into the hospital, but that cancer was really progressed, and the doctor said it was inoperable at that time. I watched my father die in the hospital. There was an NA meeting in the hospital, and I would go to that meeting at 7:00pm and talk about my father dying upstairs. Sometimes the people from that NA meeting went upstairs with me and prayed for my father. That meeting and those people got me through that experience.

I started working the steps and making amends in my early recovery, I also started working on forgiveness, especially with my mother before she passed away in 2012. Even though I had resented her throughout my life, I was able to start connecting to my mother and my sisters in Mississippi. I would call her, and I would say, "I love you, momma." And she would say, "Thank you, son." I would say again, "I love you, momma." And she'd say again, "Thank you, son." And I'd say again, "I love you, momma." And then finally she said, "I love you too." When my mother passed away I was hurting, but I was grateful that I had a relationship with her. Today, I have a great relationship with my sisters and family in Mississippi.

At the end of my addiction, I treated my grandmother and my auntie pretty bad. Me and my grandmother and auntie would go to Mississippi every year to visit my mother and my sisters. The last year before I made the decision to get clean, my aunt went to Mississippi to visit my mother, and while she was gone, me and my brothers sold all the furniture in her house for dope. And I'm talking about *everything*. We knew all the right people to sell everything to. When my grandmother and auntie got back, they sold the house, so I didn't have a house to go back to. My father was so ashamed of what I'd done to his mother that for a while I was an outcast. Me and my brothers were no longer welcome. But I finally made amends around all that. I made amends to my grandmother and my auntie, and they were real proud of me. When my grandmother and my auntie moved back to Mississippi, I went back every year to see them and my mother. They were so proud that I stayed clean, and I know they would be proud that I'm still clean today.

All those guys that were in the game started calling me Mr. Recovery. They would see me at meetings and I would always tell them, "Hey man, I've been clean five years, I've been clean ten years. I've been clean twenty years. You are still using, man; you know you can change your life. I've been working since I was clean, man; you can have this life too, man." I never had a job until I got into recovery. My first job was with St. Anthony's—that same detox that I went into, I ended up working there for five years. I looked at my intake file and it said "detox only" fifty-three times. I had fifty-three intakes at St. Anthony's detox until the last visit when it said, "St. Anthony's program." I've been clean ever since!

So recovery is possible, man. There were just a lot of things that happened in between. I met a lot of good people in Richmond and Oakland and San Francisco. This is a program of attraction, not promotion. I'm talking about recovery from the game. I'm talking about being deep in the game and knowing some people that were committed to that lifestyle. That's all they knew. That's all my father knew. That's all my brothers knew. They lived and died that game. All they knew was running gambling houses, selling weed, selling dope, hustling, fake VCR's, fake jewelry, lying, and stealing. We did what we had to do, and we were speeding off, with the money you see. We were all taking penitentiary chances for little or nothing. That's all the people around me knew, and people can only give you what they got. And so I came up with the acronym, GAME. *Good advice means everything*. G.A.M.E. I've got some good advice today, and that's why I want to talk about recovering from the game.

So yeah, they call me the Tenderloin Ambassador for Recovery because this right here, where we are, is the belly of the beast. You walk through Eddy Street and you are going to see something. Within two blocks, you are going to see somebody smoking crack, they got some foil out, you know how it is, man, that's the way it is right here. I used to shoot dope and smoke dope over at Boeddeker Park, and now we celebrate Recovery Day over there. We do rallies over there. The whole park has been remodeled. There are kids over there now. Today it's a sanctuary amidst all of this, but it used to be a devil's den. We used to go over there and just use drugs and sell drugs. I was there. I did that. I had a friend who used to just park his car and be a loan shark. People would run out of money and he would loan people money for their drugs and then collect on the first. It's different today, but you still see the same people struggling.

I made a commitment: trust God, clean house, help others. And that's my thing today. I became a Mason. Masonry has taken my recovery to another level because of the principles that are practiced. Most of all, there is charity in the lodge, located at 548 Haight Street. We have committed our kitchen to serving the community, and we have an event space called the Peacock Lounge right next-door at 552 Haight St. We own the building and rent it for private events, plus we have jazz shows the last Friday of every month. On Wednesdays we have the biggest AA meeting in the city. We do all kinds of events for the neighborhood community. We recently had the Peacock Lounge kitchen remodeled with a grant from the city, with the understanding that we will serve senior citizens every day from the kitchen. We provide scholarships for a couple schools in the city, as well.

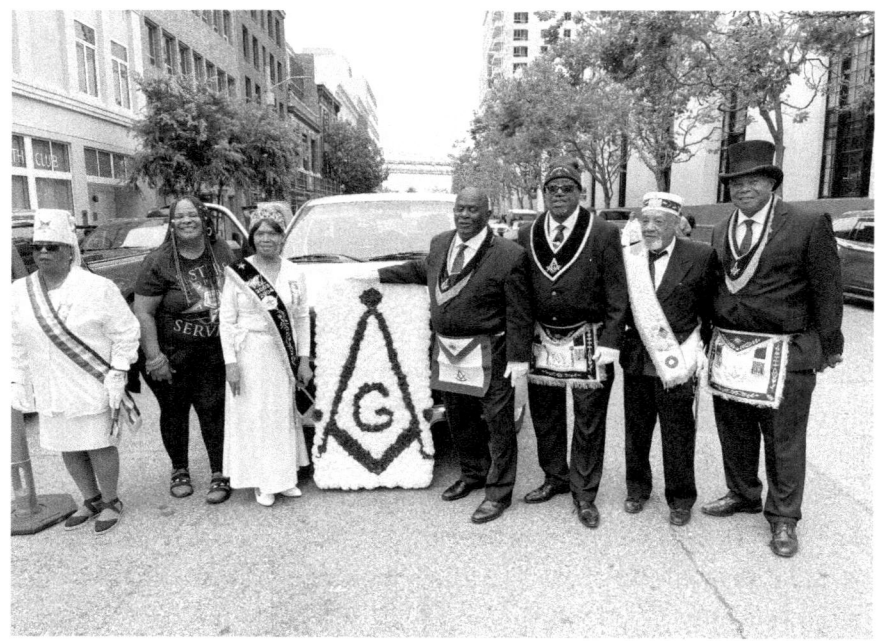

Masons and OES at 2024 Juneteenth Parade

It's been a journey. It's been a journey, man. And people still call me *Dollar Bill*. I used to say, "Dollar Bill, never worked, never will. All I do is rest and dress, make my money on the corner, everything else will do the rest. I'm sharper than a Gillette razor, got more game than Milton Bradley, if they ever dreamt about being sharper than me, they better wake up and apologize because it ain't nothin' but a dream. I do this right here with ease, I am the macaroni and I can get the cheese." I used to say all of that and believe all of that, but it was just words, just tryin' to be slick out there in the game. I used to say that I was greasier than a gas station mop. I could be wearing a grey suit one day and then three or four days later it might look like I was wearing a nice black suit. But it's the same suit, man! You know how it is when you're out there on the street, man. I ended up sleeping on the cardboard. At the end, man, I was just ripped and not caring. I had some days when I was hustling, and I had dope but I didn't have money to get a room. I would smoke on the street all night, and just pass out wherever I was at. I would just lay there, on cardboard or a blanket if I had them, and if I didn't then I didn't. That was my end, man.

Then I got clean. Today I can relate to people who come out of jail and treatment, and the struggles that they have. I can understand why some people can't sleep in a bed when they first get clean, because they got so used to sleeping on the street that sleeping on a mattress is just too much. You can't do it for a while. It's too soft. A lot of people have been programmed or institutionalized, and you gotta meet people where they are. I believe that a good counselor is not someone who has all the answers, it's someone who the ability to ask the right questions. *What do you need? How can I help you?* Those type of things.

The reason I want to write this book is because I want to let people know, even though they were or are caught up in the game, they can recover. Don't let anything hold you back. There was a time that I didn't know anything about NA or AA or any type of recovery. All I knew was the game. All I knew was hustling weed, hustling in the streets, selling junk, I knew about all that type of stuff. But the simple fact is people do recover. I want people to know, if you can run a boost crew, you can run a business. If you can run a gang, you can run a team. You've got transferable skills. If you think it can't be done, you're wrong. I know it can be done because I did it. And I know that I get more respect now as a recovering addict than I ever did when I was in the game. That's why all the guys that are still in the game call me and respect me as Mr. Recovery or the TL Ambassador for Recovery. They look at me and they say, "Oh man, that Dollar Bill right there, man, his father was a monster in the game. He comes from Richmond royalty." When I go to Richmond, they still talk about stories of the things we did way back in the day. All the fights and the gang bangin'. It's been forty years and people are still talking about this stuff. I want to let people know with this book, man, you know what, you can recover from the game. Recovery is possible. People from the Tenderloin do recover. People from Richmond do recover. People from deep East Oakland do recover. Anybody can recover. Anybody can lose that desire to use. Any addict can stop using drugs, lose the desire to use, and find a new way to live.

CHAPTER 2

International Red

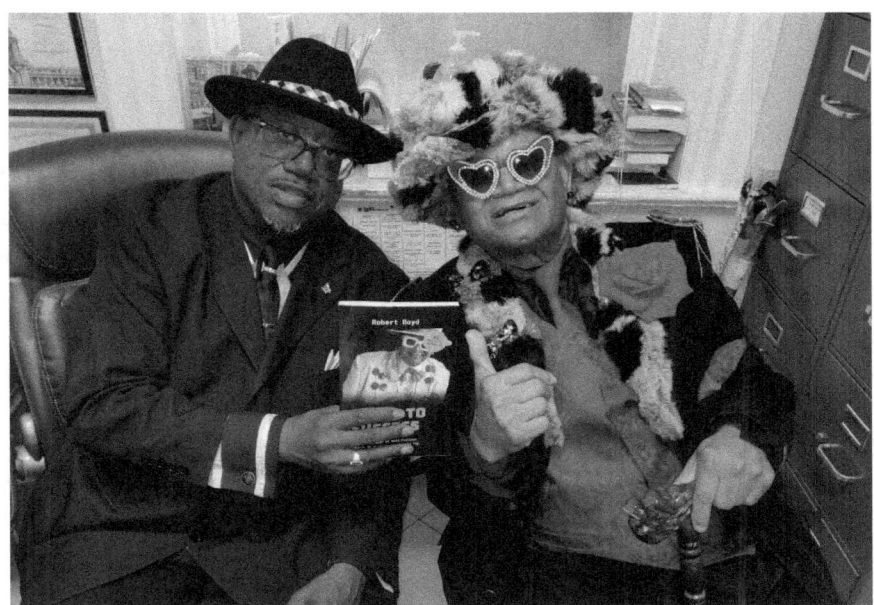

Richard and International Red with Red's book, "Socks to Success"

Richard, chatting with Mark: All right, alright! It's good to see you again, man, and it's good to enjoy another day clean. I always say it feels good to be here and it feels good to be clean. And it feels good to not focus on anything on the outside to try and fix what's going on in the inside. Anytime I think that something on the outside is going to fix what's going on in the inside, that thought is the problem. Anytime I think more sex, more dope, more clothes, the car, the job, anything, can make me feel better, that thought is the problem, man. Because I don't need anything on the outside to fix what's going on the inside.

You know, I'm glad that I have a relationship with the God of my understanding. I learned that through 12-steps recovery. It says in the AA literature, *The wider the base, the higher the point of freedom.* I think my base got really wide by trying to reach out to some of the people that I admired out there on the street back in the day, people like my father Willie Bill, and people like Fillmore Slim, and the Grandmaster Virgil Fairley. Guys like Candyman, and this one guy that I still have a relationship with that I met out on the street years ago. We weren't that close way back then. He was doing his thing and I was doing my thing and he was older than me, but I was just lookin' and he had that flair about him. His name is Robert Boyd Jr., and today we have a good relationship. We call him *International Red.* His father owned a bar and a dry cleaner business, and he was one of the first black men to have a black-owned business in the Fillmore. I met Red and Candyman when I saw them doing their thing out here in San Francisco, and all of us have been able to develop friendships over the years. I think I have a few more years of clean time than Red, but he had some clean time before as well. When I met Red again we really connected, about ten years ago. He was selling watches and CDs right outside this chicken place over on 6th Street in the Tenderloin. It has a new owner now, but back in the old days Red had a good relationship with the owners. He would set up a table, and he would put out his watches and jewelry. Red was in recovery, clean and sober—he didn't drink, he didn't use, and he would always talk about how he would go to meetings. What I admired in him was that I could see the change from then to now. It wasn't like he was selling slum and trying to sell it as real. He was selling watches, but he would give you a fair price for them. He wasn't tryin' to get one over on you. Red wouldn't try to sell you a $20 watch for $200. If Red had costume jewelry, he'd give you costume prices. Red is a fair man today, and that transformation came because of his recovery. So, when I really got to know him, he was selling his costume jewelry, watches, and CDs and he was just real cool. Whenever I would see Red, he would always stop me and say, "Hey Dollar Bill!" He still calls me Dollar Bill; I can't remember the last time he called me Richard. And I would always say, "What's up, International Red!"

Red just had his seventieth birthday, and I was able to throw him a birthday party at the Peacock Lounge. We had Fillmore Slim and his band come and play the blues, and it was really great. Of course, Red and some of his closest friends drove up in a super stretch white limo. Red is just one of the coolest guys I know, man. Red has become one of those people that I always invite to my sober events or music concerts that I help produce. Every time I put together something like a Juneteenth celebration or Black History celebration, or when my wife will do a Kwanzaa celebration, I always want to have my man Red there with me because we are just good friends like that. You never know which people you'll see in recovery that you used to see in the streets. Some of them go to jail and get clean and then you bump into them at a meeting, or some of them move out of state, they do a geographic, get clean and then move back when they get into a better situation in life. People got to go through what they gotta go through. Whatever it is, people have to do what they have to do. To me, it's many paths, one destination. But it really inspires me when it's somebody that I knew who was in the game, somebody that I knew who was out there in the streets hustling and pimpin' or whatever they were doing, and then I see them in recovery. I see them doing well, not drinking and not doing drugs, and working on themselves to be the best person they can possibly be. Red is one of those people. I am grateful to have the relationship with Red that I have today.

Five years ago, my wife had her forty-fifth birthday party and of course she invited Red. He danced with my mother-in-law; my family just loves Red. Red just has one of the most infectious personalities, everybody loves him.

Mark: While Richard was telling me about his wife's forty-fifth birthday party, Red walked into the private office that Richard and I were sitting in. Red definitely brightens up any room he walks into. Wearing an amazing three-piece white, gold, and brown suit with a matching hat sitting on top of his bright red curly hair, he completed his outfit with an antique wooden walking cane with a gold eagle's head as the handle. International Red is the very definition of "cool."

Red: Hey, hey, hey, hey, hey!

Richard: Speak of the devil! And entering my office right now, is the legendary Robert Boyd Jr., San Francisco's very own International Red! Hey Red, man, tell us what's going on, man.

Red: So how do we do this, man? What do you need from me, Mr. Dollar Bill?

Richard: Well, Red, as you know, I invited you over today because I want you to be in my book, *Recovering From The Game*. I was just telling Mark here how we have been close over the last ten years.

Red: Well, this is International Red, and I was born and raised in San Francisco but I went all over the country since I was six years old. Most of my life I was in the game traveling the country, mostly under the influence. But I have gotten a second chance at a first-class life. When I got clean is when I really started to live. I *thought* I was living before that. People think they are living when they are in the game and living the fast life, but really you ain't lived until you have lived clean and sober, and then you're living a good life. You understand what I'm sayin', man?

Richard: So, Red how old were you when you got into the life?

Red: Into the fast life? Oh, I was sixteen. You see what happened was, I was in high school. My cousin was already out in the streets. I didn't know she was in the streets, but when she came by my mother's house out in Pacifica, she was in a brand-new car. She was driving a brand-new MG sports car. My cousin came by and she was wearing all this fancy jewelry and she had all these fancy clothes on. Back then my cousin was telling everybody that she was a model and that she was modeling out of Vegas, New York, and LA. But one day I saw my cousin out in the Tenderloin. She was walking down Eddy Street where we are right now, actually. This was back in 1967, back when everything was happening. So, I saw my cousin and she ran up to me and told me not to tell anybody what she was doing. That's the day I found out she was whoring and hustlin' men. I told her I wouldn't tell anybody, but she had to teach me the game. I wanted to be a pimp, boom-boom. I had been seeing pimps riding their fancy cars up and down the streets in the Tenderloin and I wanted me some of that. I hadn't gotten my feet wet yet, and I wanted to make it happen, you see. I told my cousin that I wanted this hot cheerleader number at my high school that didn't want nothin' to do with me to be one of my girls, but my cousin told me that I didn't want that. She told me that I didn't want no fancy girls, that I needed to find a woman whose self-esteem ain't tight. She told me to get a girl that nobody wanted instead. So, what happened was, I went and did what my cousin said. I went to school, befriended a girl, walked around with her, held hands with her for about a week. Everybody was laughing at me and her, but I didn't trip because I had a goal. I told the girl, 'Me and you, we goin' to the top. You're going to be a star; we're going to go to the Tenderloin and we're going to make it happen.' We ran away to the Tenderloin, but I didn't have her more than a month before one of those fancy pimps with jewelry and a brand-new Cadillac knocked me. He took my girl. But my cousin told me, "Don't worry about it. You did what you're supposed to do. You got your feet wet; you turned somebody out and you got somebody in the game. Now you know how it goes. All you have to do is take your time and get yourself a car and hold on to your money." My cousin gave me little pointers in the game to get me started.

Richard: How did you get the name *International Red*?

Red: I got the name *International Red* when I was up there in Seattle. When I went to Seattle I was just called *Red*, and I had a massage parlor up there, right. I had women working in the Seattle massage parlor, and I would go across up to Canada on the train every weekend with this cat named Cadillac. Cadillac and I would go to Gastown where the girls used to dance, and then I'd bring a couple girls from Gastown back down to Seattle and they'd work in my massage parlor. I was going back and forth every weekend, so everybody started calling me International Red. Not because I was goin' to Paris, or Rome, or London like Cadillac did. They started calling me International Red in the '70s because I was going back and forth between Canada and America. Back in the day some of the boys would call me *Cross Country Red* or *Fast Red* but I liked *International Red*, so I stuck with it, and I carry that name today.

Richard: So tell me Red, how did you make the decision to come into recovery after being so deep in the game and knowin' all the players in the game? Because I used to see you out there, man, you know, you were poppin' back when I saw you out there.

Red: See, what happened was I came out of the joint in 1983, right. I was up in Tacoma, Washington, McNeil Island, and that's where I met CB and a couple other players. I told them, man, when I get out of here, man, I'm serious, I'm not going to be drinking or using anymore. I'm going to take care of my business. I'm still going to be in the game, I'm a pimp, I'm a player. I'm going to do all the things I got to do but I ain't goin' to get high, I ain't touchin' nothin'. And that's what I did. I got out, I didn't change anything about my life, but I didn't get high. I stopped gettin' high, man. For ten years, I didn't get high. But I was still in the game as far as working after hours, havin' hoes, prostitutes, doin' all that stuff. So many people would ask me how I was doing all the same things, runnin' the girls, hustlin', but not drinking, and not getting high. I was runnin' with Pretty Boy, and he was on dope. People that knew I was sober would tell me what I was doin' wasn't cool, that it didn't make no sense. But why would I stop? I had a Cadillac, I had a Benz, I had five cars and I had a house out in Clear Lake. I told everybody, "Look man, I'm doin' good, you can't tell me nothin'." I wasn't going to listen to nobody. Like I said, I had ten years clean. But then my mother got sick, and that was hard on me. One night I went to an after-hours party depressed, and I just took a hit of that blow. I'd been ten years clean when I hit that blow, and the next thing you know I'm drinking. Six months later I lost five cars, I lost the house in Clear Lake, I'm on the street in front of the liquor store, dirty and tore up over on 6th and Jessie Street. I was tore up, and people were taking pictures of me and talking about me. Eventually I went to my cousin's. I was in a messed-up place, man. My sister and the rest of my family wouldn't have anything to do with me once I started drinking again. I didn't have any more money, and when you don't have money, people don't want to have anything to do with you. But when I went to my cousin, the same cousin that helped me get into the game, she's the one that helped me get clean. She wasn't even clean, but she was the one who told me to go to meetings. She helped me get a new ID, she helped me get on welfare, and then she had me go to Glide Church and join all the programs I had to join. One day at a time, I was able to get a year sober with my cousin's help. This was back in 1998. I went to AA meetings, I got the Big Book, and I just did what I had to do. One day at a time. The year 1998 was when I learned I couldn't do it on my own.

Richard: So how long have you been clean now, Red?

Red: Twenty-seven years now.

Richard: Twenty-seven years. So you had ten years, then you relapsed for six months, and now you got twenty-seven.

Red: Right. I don't know my exact clean date, but I know it was around my birthday. It was in the beginning of summer of 1998.

Richard: You know, I take my hat off to people who just went to meetings and were able to get clean and stay clean. Because I couldn't do it. I had to go to treatment.

Red: The first time, when I got my ten years, I was doing a lot of treatments when I was in the joint, in '83. And when I got out, I didn't have a support system. I was on the road. I was in Denver, I was in Albuquerque, Phoenix, Las Vegas, I was all over with pimps and players and people that were getting' high. For ten years I didn't touch it, but eventually it got me. Today, I know how dangerous all this is, so today I don't want to be around anybody that is getting high. If I see someone getting high around me, I get away as quick as I can. No joke, man. Because sometimes you don't have any more recoveries in you. The older you get, the more progressive the disease is, so you can't count on another recovery. You don't want to lose what you got. You just say, this is it and I'm taking this to the grave. And today, man, I try to be as humble as I can. I don't go around tellin' everybody how many years clean I have anymore. Even to this day there are some people that don't know how much clean me I got. They don't need to know everything I got goin on.

When I got clean the second time, I didn't get around the people that were in the game. I got with people that were out of the game. Like Fillmore Slim, he used to be in the game but he left all that behind. I want to surround myself with people that want to live clean and do live clean. I can't blame anybody for what they used to do. All that matters is what we got goin' on now. When I got into the Fillmore Bay Area Media Group, there was a bunch of us that used to be in the game but we had all cleaned ourselves up. We'd go to City Hall and we'd be doin' positive things and trying to keep things going. That kept all of us active in our recovery.

Richard: Yeah, I remember when you started that Fillmore Media Group. So, who was in that Fillmore Media Group? How many years ago was that?

Red: About ten years ago. Yeah, it was Ace Washington, we had Rico Hamilton, there was Ken Johnson, Charie Walker, Candyman, and CB was all in. There were about ten or fifteen of us. And it was cool. We were trying to make things happen. As black people we were trying to get the young kids computers for school and teach them how to dress up and get jobs. We really wanted to make a difference in our community. And from that group I tried to start another group which didn't really go anywhere, but then I got into the group with you.

Richard: That's right. West Coast Entertainment.

Red: West Coast Entertainment Association. That's been a lot of fun. Richard, you had me speak at your first Recovery Day a few years back. I was your first speaker, and that was great, too. So like I said, I don't take my recovery for granted anymore. You never know how much time you have here, right. And you got to look at people that are older than you and doing good. You have to take a look at them and take a page out of their book. You gotta take that page and compare it to what it is that you are doing, and just keep moving on. And like Del Seymour once said, "You can be in the Tenderloin, but you don't let the Tenderloin make you, you make the Tenderloin. You can still be strong." We see all those people on the ground, but what Del Seymour said inspired me to stay off the ground. I don't want to be down and out with them.

Richard: So, Red, I know I have seen you in some pictures with a few mayors over the years. How many mayors have stood with you over the years? I know you were declared one of the best dressed in San Francisco.

Red: Oh, Mayor Willie Brown, he gave me that. Willie actually gave Smiley the key to the city and a couple of other plaques. I told Willie that Smiley is my mentor, and that Smiley actually passed me the torch. So, one day when I saw Willie Brown, I said, 'Hey man, you didn't officially give me the title but I'm holding the title of best dressed in San Francisco and nobody else is doin' like I'm doin' it.' And Willie said, 'Yeah man, you're holdin' it down.' And the reason why I say this is because I was there for Smiley. Everybody was always tryin' to put Smiley down. Smiley never got clean, right. He never got clean and sober. But one thing about Smiley, he was a functioning addict. He could maneuver and do everything. He could dress, talk, walk, and dance like no other.

This is what happened, this is a true story. I was riding with Pretty Boy; we were on Broadway in San Francisco, and this lady had an art gallery. One day I went into this art gallery and I saw Smiley's picture in there. Smiley was sick at the time, and I said, 'Wait a minute! You know, that's my partner Smiley, that's his picture.' And the woman told me that she had been looking for Smiley for years. They had sold the painting of Smiley, and they wanted to give him some money but they couldn't find him. I told the woman that I'd come by tomorrow and I'd bring Smiley with me. But Pretty Boy didn't want to take me over to Smiley's. No, he wanted to hate on Smiley. "No man, I ain't taking you over to Smiley's!" "Come on Pretty Boy, I'll pay you. Why do you want to act like that, man? You shouldn't be hatin', man. Smiley is a good dude, man." "Oh, man, I used to smoke with Smiley. I know he ain't nothin'."

I said, "Why you like this, man? I look up to Smiley. I kick it with Smiley, and he taught me a lot of game, man." I convinced Pretty Boy to help me pick up Smiley the next day. So, the next day Pretty Boy and I picked up Smiley and we took him to the art gallery. They gave Smiley $600. Then the gallery owner threw Smiley a birthday party, and the people that attended the birthday party helped Smiley reconnect with some old friends. A lot of good things came from that painting and that birthday party. But anyway, to make a long story short, they had the party, they did all that, and I was there when all that went down. I supported Smiley, man. I was always in his corner. That's what real friends do, man. You gotta be there for your partners. You don't abandon them when they're down. You gotta be there for your partners, good or bad. And Pretty Boy, you know, that's why he never had good luck. Because he always wanted to hate on people. I always told Pretty Boy, "Man, there ain't no room for hate, man. That's why you ain't got no love." You got to give credit where credit is due. If a dude is better than you, if he's got a finer woman or his catch hand is better, you gotta give him that respect. Acknowledge that. Don't hate on that, man. That's what I was trying to tell Pretty Boy back then.

Richard: Well, Red, man, the legendary International Red, I just want to thank you for volunteering to be a part of my book. I want to thank you for telling your story and thank you for being my friend, especially for the past ten-plus years. When I thought about writing this book, you were the first person that I knew I had to interview. That's why you were the first person I introduced to Mark. I really appreciate you taking the time out of your day and telling us your amazing story man. Thank you, Red.

Red: Well yeah, man, I can tell it like it is because a lot of people don't understand, man. They don't realize that some people don't tell the truth, don't do things to really inform you. And that's what I try to tell people. I say, "No, you gotta realize that people are going to tell you things, but if you don't have the experience, life is going to be different from what all those people told you." A lot of people will tell you things that happened years ago. When I was getting my information in the pool hall or in the coffee shop with those older cats, we were doing the same thing at the same time. We weren't talking about old war stories, twenty or thirty years ago. Today a lot of guys will be talkin' to other cats, sittin' at the bus stop, talking about what they did twenty years ago. When somebody gives you information on something that is going on right now, that's a different thing. And back when I was a youngster, when the pool halls were open, the old cats used to talk to young people. There wasn't this generation gap that we have right now. When that crack came out, there was a generation gap that started. The youngsters that were sellin' dope to the older cats lost respect for the older cats, so the younger people don't listen to them anymore. Right, to this day, a lot of cats tell me, "Man, you look good and I'll listen to you. But those other older cats, when they try to talk to me, man, I don't listen to them. But I know you know what's goin' on." And I always say, "Man, I know what's goin' on in the streets, but I ain't got time to talk to you about the streets. Let's talk about recovery and how to stay out of jail!"

CHAPTER 3

The Candyman

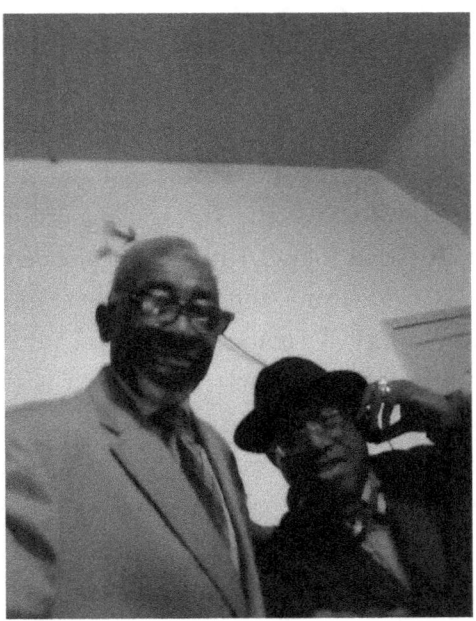

Richard: So, Candyman, I'm glad that you decided to interview for my book, *Recovering From The Game*. You are one of the first men I met coming out here to San Francisco that was already in the game. You know International Red, Mac Breed, you know Mac Edge, you know all my guys from Richmond. I know that you came out here from New York, and we all ended up in San Francisco goin' to the Players Ball at the Bayview Opera House. Every time I see something going on as far as the Players Ball, and stuff like that, I always see you, Candyman. I know you were having some health issues recently, but it looks like you are back. So I am glad you are here and I am glad you are healthy. When you had your heart attack, I visited you in the hospital because you have been such a role model for me over the years. Man, as far as bein' in the game, deep in the game, bein' in recovery, having family in recovery, you've been such a role model for me. I know your daughter, Candice, is big in recovery, and I think her mother just celebrated twenty-five years. So, Candyman, I just want you to be part of the book, man. This is your recovery, this is your time, and thank you for your participation. I really, really do appreciate you. I want to introduce y'all to Dejenney Davis, a.k.a. the Candyman!

Candyman: Thank you, brother. Thank you for that little endorsement. Yeah, you know, recovery is when you have a made-up mind. And what we've been through in our life, whether it was using drugs or something else, it was a way of life for us, right. And most of the people we really looked up to, guys like you and me, those people were in the game. Most of those people used drugs. We come from a drug culture. We came up in that. It had a different effect back then than it has today. The world has changed. But one thing that stays the same, anytime you use any kind of mind-altering substance, sometimes you don't make the best decisions in your life. And guys like you and me, we've been through a lot of things, man. I've been to and have lived through penitentiaries like San Quentin. And when you get out, you get on a bus that drops you off in the middle of the Tenderloin and you got $200 in your pocket. The whole thing feels rigged to make you go back out. Same thing in New York, man. The system knows what time the buses come from each penitentiary, or wherever else you are coming from. The penitentiary knows where the bus is taking you, and those bad places are just waiting for you and your money, man.

Richard: What year did you come out here from New York?

Candyman: I'm originally from Tulsa, Oklahoma, but we came out to California when I was five years old. Raised in the Fillmore District, but I lived half my adult life in New York City. All of my twenties, thirties, and forties, you see. There was a time in my life where I wouldn't have left New York City to go to heaven, because New York was the place to be.

When I was coming up and getting into the game, Boedecker Park, here in San Francisco, was a bowling alley. The police station across the street from the park was a numbers yard. Gambling, you see. Everything on both sides of Eddy Street, from Van Ness to Mason, was titty bars, man. At the same time this was going on, Vietnam was goin' on too. And every single branch of the military, goin' or comin' from Vietnam, was comin' through Treasure Island. So back then all you would see was a lot of action. A lot of money, 24/7, man. It was happening out here, man. And while the war was goin' on, you had the Haight and Ashbury scene goin' on too. Then you had the Black Panthers. And then you had the Hells Angels. All of this was happening during the same time period. It was a unique time in history. It was a unique time to be alive. There was a lot of money, and we were young and buying Cadillacs, tailor-made suits, alligator shoes, jewelry, we had it all, man. We were just teenagers, man! We used to have a $1500 club. You have $1500 in one pocket and your spending money in another pocket. It was nothin' for us to carry $3000 or $4000 at all times. This is how San Francisco was for some of us back then. Then I went back to New York.

Richard: How old were you when you went back to New York?

Candyman: I was about twenty years old, and I really got introduced to the real game when I went back to New York. New York is the fastest, biggest, baddest city in the world. The capital of everything. I lived in Harlem for a bit, but mostly I lived in the Village. I lived in Brooklyn for a time, the Bronx, Staten Island, I lived in all five boroughs by the time I was done. I got my GED in Elmira Correctional Facility in Upstate New York. That's forty miles from Montreal. You salute two flags when you are way up there, man. And they are mad at you when they send you all the way up there, man. It starts snowing in the middle of July. It's way up in the mountains. When I was up there, a lot of guys would tell me that those mountains out there are the incest capital of the world. They were killin' inmates up there back then. If you are coming up there, especially if you are coming out of New York City, you gotta get a hotel room and stay the weekend. It's far up in the mountains. People were breakin' in, raping people's daughters, man, it was a mess goin' on up there. They were killing inmates and burying them. It was really goin' down up there, man. You see, New York has some notorious prisons, and I've been to all of them. I've been to Sing Sing, Elmira, Attica, and Comstock. I got into a couple stabbings myself in Comstock. But then you have Rikers Island, and Rikers is a whole other thing, man. It's not the state's penitentiary, it's the city's penitentiary. And each borough of New York has its own house. Like the Brooklyn House of Detention, then you have the Bronx House of Detention, Queens House of Detention, Staten Island House of Detention, and Manhattan Island House of Detention. And the Manhattan Island House of Detention is called *the Tombs*. I've been to all of them houses. But after being institutionalized for so long, eventually, you want to change things. I wanted to change things. It ain't been easy, but like a lot of things in life, eventually, you gotta make a change.

Wakin' up, dead broke. The worst feeling in the world is to wake up broke. But some of us got into that comfort zone, wakin' up broke, tryin' to find that money and paying for the hit by the day. You always find a way to get that money because you need that hit. Back in the old days, only a certain kind of person used drugs, but now it seems like the entire society is using drugs of some kind, it's a problem. Today, people would rather take a hit than pay down on a place to stay. You start realizing that all those hits you take in order to make your troubles go away, you start to realize that the troubles will always come back and you have to deal with them eventually. The hit only lasts so long, and it's never long enough. But if you don't face your troubles, those troubles will be there until the day you die.

Richard: Do you remember the year you came back to San Francisco from New York?

Candyman: I came back here after my baby sister died, so around 2004. Before that I was all over the country, man. I've been in jail in forty-eight cities and fourteen states, man. I was in and out of jail doin' those skid bits.

Richard: When did you meet International Red?

Candyman: I met Red back in the early '60s, maybe back in 1962. You see, back in the day there were pool halls and clubs everywhere in San Francisco. We had clubs in Fillmore, North Beach, and Chinatown. There was this club in Chinatown, Rickshaw. Now that was a good catch spot. The ladies that went there were top notch.

Richard: What's the deepest you ever been, Candyman? How many women were working for you at one time?

Candyman: Man, I normally had maybe three or four girls, but I liked having my thieves. I liked my bank robbers. Rane was a bank robber. We all knew Rane here in the Tenderloin. She was a good bank robber. I think I was eighteen and Rane was seventeen at the time. Her stepmom used to help us out from time to time. I would always teach my girls how to pick pocket. I wanted them to find as many ways as possible to take that money from those men. One of my girls, Laura, she was one of my best thieves. One day she showed up with $27,000 and just threw it on my lap. No questions asked, she just threw down that money. Laura was a good girl, man.

Richard: So Laura and Rane, they were part of your boost crew. They were boostin' for you back then as well.

Candyman: Well, yeah, they were boostin', man. They were cold with it, man. When I first met Laura, I had a blue and white Cadillac. I think it was a '73 Cadillac, and Laura sold it for some dope. She sold it to Code Chief and that's down over in Hayes Valley, so I went over to him and he let me buy my car back. I think I got the car back for $400.

I got clean and sober the first time over in Dallas, Texas, in 2004. 'Cause I came back to California through Dallas, right. I got sober in Dallas in 2004, and then six months later I came back to California. For the first couple years I lived with one of my family members, and then in 2007 I got an apartment here in San Francisco. I have been in that same apartment ever since, but I am about to move in a week or so.

You know, when you start seein' the behavior of the people that you associate with and you are doing drugs and acting out with them, you just can't take none of that back. After a while you start to see that there's no excuse to do drugs. It took me a while to see what I was doing. I would always start usin' again because I was right here in the Tenderloin. Everybody I knew was out using. The ones that weren't using, they're still not using to this day. To be honest with you, I started using almost immediately after I got back to San Francisco in 2005. As soon as I got back I reconnected with one of my best friends on this earth, whose name is Connie Hill. We came up in New York together. I knew Connie was in San Francisco, so you know I was going to look for Connie. So, Connie and I reconnected, and we would do our drugs together and run with our girls. Things escalated to the point where I was a full-fledged crack addict. I was not happy with it. And of course, you don't meet women when you are in this kind if state. Nobody wants anything to do with a crack addict. The thing about it, man, is once you go back into that addiction, it will take you back to that bad behavior.

The life that we used to live is nothin' like it is today. The world is so different today from the world I knew when I was comin' up. The whole system of the game has changed. Back in the old days, we had respect in the streets. There were certain things we didn't let youngsters do that the kids are allowed to do now. We used to run these young kids on home if they were in the wrong part of town, man. We'd tell these kids to get their ass to school or we'd tell them to go home. We'd run the young girls home if they were too young. But the streets don't have that order now. Now, these new cats in the game will see a young kid and put a pipe in that kid's mouth. They'll put a spike in their arm."

Richard: So, your oldest baby's mother got clean. She has almost thirty years clean now.

Candyman: Yeah, that sounds about right.

Richard: The first time I saw you clean was back when you were doing the Fillmore Bay Area Media Group. Tell me about that.

Candyman: Yeah, that's right. I had just got clean again in 2012 when we started that. Back then I was having a hard time staying clean, because when I would run out of money people would just give me whatever I wanted. Women would stop by my place wanting a safe place to use and then before you know it, I was back to smokin' again. This was a tough time because by this time I had acknowledged that I was doing wrong. I might not even have dope on my mind, but someone would always come and knock on my door and it would start all over again. So, this particular night, it was December 28, 2012, I got a girl stayin' with me. I had this girl and this other woman named Fifi at my place, and they wanted to go get something. So, I called a girl that I knew would deliver what they wanted. I had to go to the ATM, and I was going to get $40, but the girls hit me up for $80. When I got back to the house, I just didn't feel comfortable. Things didn't feel right. I took a good look at myself, and I looked at the women that were in my apartment, and I knew right then and there that I could do better than what I was doing. I could do better than this. I just decided then and there that I didn't want any more of that.

Two days later I went out on New Year's. I had a bit of money on me that night. I think I had about $2000 in cash on me, and I also had a check for another $1000. I was getting ready to go into my building, and here come the girls again. These are girls that I used to mess with, but I told them I didn't want anything from them anymore. Then, when I got ready to open my front door, another girl that I used to get with happened to be walking down the hallway in front of my door. Well, she also just happened to have a purse full of money on her and two or three pipes ready to go with dope in them, right. But I didn't want any of it, man. I didn't want one hit of it. All I knew is that I had to get into my apartment and close the door before another lady decided to stop by my place. I didn't know how much more temptation I was going to be able to take that night. If one more person had stopped by my place that night, I don't know if I ever would have gotten sober.

Richard: So, you're saying you got clean at the beginning of 2013? And then you stayed clean for nine years, til 2022.

Candyman: So, yeah, til about 2022. There was a girl that stayed in the complex I have been living at. There are a lot of senior citizens like me staying in this building. She and I would get together once in a while and mess around. She was using drugs, but I wouldn't use drugs with her. But eventually, I started using with her. Right around my birthday, she handed me the pipe and I took that hit. I was so weak, and I just took it. That was in January of 2022. I wouldn't do it again for another six months. I was so mad at myself. Then I'd go from every six months to once every ninety days, and then I got to the point where I just had to let it go again. I just don't want to go back to that ever again. Once you get clean and sober, you don't ever want to see any of it again. You don't want to be associated with that junk.

Richard: Going back to the Fillmore Media Group, man. I used to see you and Red hangin' out. What happened with the Fillmore Media Group? Because it was goin' good for a minute. And I knew you were all doing advocacy work and you were focused on getting rights for African Americans, people not getting services in the Fillmore, helping out the kids and talking to the press and holding rallies for the African American community in the Bay Area. And you had all those guys that were in the game. It was you, Red, CB, Rodie Mac, Willie P, there were so many of you at one time.

Candyman: Yeah, well, we were trying to do something in the entertainment field.

Richard: Yeah, but you were also pimps and players and you were deep into that game, man.

Candyman: Yeah, we were living that fast life back then. Well, man, things change. I have seen the world change twice. I mean overnight. The world changed when crack cocaine came out, and during the covid pandemic. You see, I left here for New York in 1976 and back out here in '78, and by then everybody was talking about freebase. I would see dudes that had been driving Cadillacs and wearing tailor-made suits in '76, they weren't doin' it the way they used to when I came back in '78. Everything had changed. All those dudes that had had money were now flat broke and struggling because of crack. Everyone was talkin' about freebase and using freebase, and I knew I never wanted to mess with that stuff. It ruined everybody. But I was here only four or five months before I was using freebase. The first night I used crack, I think I spent maybe $500 or $600, and I would have spent more but they just cut me off. They wouldn't sell me any more that night. Maybe they ran out. Maybe they felt sorry for me.

It ain't never been the same since crack hit. All of the sudden all the fathers were gone in all the black neighborhoods, and I don't think anything has ever gotten better since that time. And then when the pandemic hit. Crack and the pandemic, man. Those are the two things I've seen that changed the world overnight, never to go back. We are living in a whole different world today, and I don't think a lot of people want to admit that to themselves. Crack and the pandemic have devastated this country, man. They devastated the world. I have seen a lot in my life, man. But I ain't seen nothin' as bad as crack. And now you got this drug, fentanyl. I've heard horror stories on it, man. I've seen horror stories on it. People are tellin' me now that you can rub that stuff on you and OD. Who ever heard of something like that happening? That's bad, man. That's a society that's goin' buck wild. These are some crazy times, man. You have to careful of everything you do or say these days. And I see a lot of people that can't understand what's really goin' on. So they drown themselves in alcohol and these drugs on the streets. They drown themselves in these mind-altering things in order to get away from this world that has them so confused and scared. But when they come back to reality, all their money is gone. That's when the devil gets you, man. The devil gets you while you are away from reality, while you are on that booze and those street drugs. When you wake up, all you want to do is to keep getting high. That's all that's on your mind. "F" everything else.

Richard: You named your daughter Candice after your name, the Candyman, right? How did you feel when Candice got clean?

Candyman: She has ten years now. I was so glad when she got clean. You see, I had made the first move back then. I was clean when Candice decided to get clean. Once I got clean, a lot of my family decided to get clean. Her momma always clean. Candice has never looked back. And my granddaughters got clean too. My granddaughters ain't looked back.

Richard: And when you had your heart attack a few years ago, was it from your relapse?

Candyman: I got a heart valve, they put in an artificial heart valve. That's what I have now. But also, when I put all that gold in my mouth, I knew I was going to have a problem. I got sick from all my gold teeth, so I had to have all that taken out. I got an infection from my gold teeth, so they took twenty-four of my teeth out and then I had an operation.

Richard: So it had nothing to do with all the drugs you were doing throughout your life?

Candyman: Well, I'm sure the drugs didn't help. I'm sure the drugs had something to do with it. I mean, over a period of time, all those drugs and all that booze is going to have some effect on your body, right? But the minute you stop all that mess, man, this is the best high in the world being sober.

Richard: When I used to see you out front of Yoshi's, Red was clean. Because Red had already been clean for a long time back then. But I used to see you, Red, and Pretty Boy, you were clean then. So, most of the time when I would see you around, you were clean. But when you were using, I just didn't see you. I never saw any of what you are talking about. I would see you when you were clean and you were doing your thing but when you relapsed, I didn't see you. You were gone.

Candyman: See, what I did in the 2000s is I would get messed up with some girl for a while and after a while I'd detox myself. I never went to hospitals or anything. But one day, I was visiting our boy Clarence at a clean and sober house, and this woman talked about how she had twenty-two years sober but one day, she went there. She relapsed, just like I did when I had some time. And she said that she went all those years but not enough days.

Richard: Too many years but not enough days. Man, ain't that the truth, man.

Candyman: She had twenty-two years and all of a sudden, she just fell off. And she said she had to start her clean date all over again. After twenty-two years she had to start all over again, man. That's some hard stuff, man.

I thought about how much time I have wasted throughout my life. None of it made any sense. It's all just a damn shame, man. It's stupid, it's ignorant, and I don't ever want to relive what I've been through. That was all my choice. So, I made a choice not to do it. One day at a time, I choose not to do it. I still got a couple young women that have my number and still try to drop by my door. I have to keep tellin' them not to come near my house, man. That's the rule, man. If you are into dope, don't come knocking on my door. It's that simple, man. Now, I'm not rude to anyone. I'm not going to cuss anyone out, but I will let them know they ain't welcome at my place as long as they are wrapped up in all that booze and dope, man. I don't put up with no nonsense anymore, man.

Richard: Yeah, Candyman, you know you got into that movie, *The Last Black Man in San Francisco*. You have had interesting experiences, Candyman.

Candyman: You see, I came up as a youngster sellin' weed down at Trees Pool Hall back in the Fillmore days. Back in the Mo. Nobody called it the Western Addition; we called it *the Mo*. I would bounce around all the hotels. Me and little Butch used to sit up there and sell dope when we were youngsters. I used to hang with a lot of cats like Butch. Local boys that would live in their momma's basements their whole life, man. They'd drive their Cadillacs and I used to say to these boys, it don't take much for a local boy to win a hometown decision. Put that Cadillac on that white line and see how long you last. If you're just a local boy doin' alright in your hometown, go across country and do it. That's where it counts, man.

Richard: Oh, you're sayin' take that Cadillac and put in on that white line and drive it across the country. Make your own way.

Candyman: I used to tell Butch and all those other local boys, you are a pimp lookalike, man. You are a pimp impersonator, living in your momma's basement.

Richard: Oh, man, Candyman, I just want to thank you because I've been watching you, man, for a number of years. I know your daughter well; we are good friends. I've been watching you for the last couple of decades, you know, you and I have been good friends all this time.

Candyman: Well, man, this is just an extension of the game, man. The game is still goin' on, man. You see, one of the reasons why I moved away from the Fillmore Media Group is because I had a chance to work with a cat named Speedy Woods. Me and Speedy Woods got together with the archbishop. The archbishop started to open the doors to the church so we could have community meetings. And some of the people in the Fillmore Group and I stopped meeting eye to eye on some things, and I just wasn't goin' for what they wanted to do anymore. Things change, man. Nothing is forever. Me and the archbishop used to go to City Hall to demand what we wanted, back when London Breed was the supervisor of District 5. London had my back. London was from the Fillmore's OC Project, and London got Willie Brown to speak at some of my events back in the day.

Richard: So, you know London Breed's family, right? You know her father and her brother, you know all of them, right?

Candyman: Yeah, I know London's whole family really well. I helped London with her first campaign [for San Francisco mayor]. I helped when everyone was tryin' to remove her. I went off on all those people that were tryin' to get rid of her and some of them backed right off of her. London is family to me, man.

Richard: Man, this has been so much fun, Candyman. Again, I want to thank you for being here and giving us everything you have today. But I just want to ask you, Candyman, what your ending message is as far as, bein' in the game, and now bein' in recovery?

Candyman: Right, well, if you use, you lose.

CHAPTER 4

Salahudin Akbar a.k.a. "Sixth Street Sid"

Alright, y'all, so now I'm proud to be speaking with a good friend of mine who came up from Los Angeles. We ran into each other using in the Tenderloin, specifically on 6th Street. At the end I went all the way down to sellin' the Coalition on Homelessness newspaper, *Street Sheet,* and hustling on the street for nickels and dimes. You know how some people start at the bottom and work their way to the top? Well, I started up top sellin' dope, and ended at the bottom, strung out and tore up. I came out here trying to conquer the world and ended up sleeping in doorways, man. And on that way down, I met my good friend Mr. Akbar, I always called him Sid, and I always saw him on 6th Street so I called him *6th Street Sid*. Before my recovery I used to run around town, losing or breaking my pipe. I always ended up smoking with Sid because he managed to hang onto his pipe. I would try taking Sid's pipe from time to time, but that never went over too well.

As soon as Sid saw me clean, he got clean too. Recovery is a program of attraction rather than promotion. I have twenty-nine years now, and he's right behind me. We both ended up going through the St. Anthony's program. We actually came into the program together, and then I stayed, and he went back out to do a little more research and came back again. But I want to let Sid tell his story on all that.

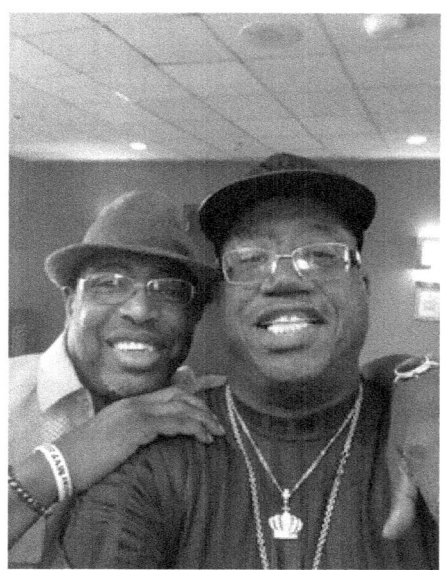

Salahudin Akbar, a.k.a. "Sixth Street Sid," and Dollar Bill

Akbar: Yeah, I've been knowin' Richard for quite a while, as a matter of fact. Three decades, plus. In the process of growing and developing, I had no idea that the devastation I was experiencing in that lifestyle of active addiction was going to be the catalyst for me helping others change their lives. God knows exactly where He wants us to be, way ahead of us knowing. That experience I had of active addiction prepared me for the work I ended up doing for over two decades. I'm no longer officially working as a provider, but in some capacity I still do that work, because some people still think that I'm a treatment specialist and call me for referrals. I did a referral for a person just last week, because I still have connections with people that do the work.

At the time I was hopeless and helpless, and I couldn't see past my life without some form of a chemical. Whether it was crack, alcohol, weed, or something else to make me feel differently than how I felt. How I felt is not what I wanted to, but I didn't know any way of changing how I felt other than trying another substance. This went on for years, and it kept getting worse even when I had ideas and expectations and hopes that it would be better this time. It never worked out like that. That experience is what helped me help others: and understanding that as much as you would like for it to get better, it's never going to get better for you if you try to use something outside of yourself to change the way you feel on the inside. That's my reality. Now I've got a productive life: I pretty much do what I wanna do when I wanna do it, with the lovely lady in my life, my wife.

I want to say thank you to Richard for asking me to do this interview. This wasn't even planned. I happened to call a friend of mine, right, to see if I could get him to take me out to lunch. That didn't work, but I'm here doin' an interview about the experience that we had together, an experience that we survived while so many people didn't. Richard can tell you we've both been told that we should be seeing a therapist for some of the things that we actually witnessed in active addiction.

Richard: I do have a therapist.

Akbar: Oh trust me, I saw a therapist in early recovery. I don't see a therapist now, but I got a mentor, I got a coach, you know, I got people that support me in my thought process.

I'm tellin' you, I used drugs from the East Coast to up north in Washington state. And I have a funny story for you on this. I was on my way up to Alaska with the idea that I was going to work one of those fishing boats, get paid a lump sum of money at the end of the job, and then buy a whole lot of drugs. I had it all planned out on how I was going to be, I was goin' to be The Man when I returned. Everything was lined up— I had my sleeping bag, I had clothes—but man, I messed around on the way to the boat. It wasn't God's plan for me to get on that fishing boat in Alaska. You see, somebody offered me a hit of crack before I got to the boat, and the boat doesn't wait on you if you are a little late. When I look back on that experience and I think, man, how did I end up here, man? But let me tell you, I smoked dope and I was out of control. Dope controlled me, thoroughly. I couldn't resist the impulse to try and get a hit. I look back on that story and thank God I missed that boat. Because I can see myself in Alaska just trying to figure it all out. How was I going to get me a hit? That was my reality back then. I was totally consumed by active addiction. It was all my waking thoughts, and I never went to sleep. No, I passed out, and dope was the last thing I did before I passed out. One time, I passed out with a crack pipe in my hand, and when I woke up the next morning I had gouged my hand squeezing that crack pipe. It took three months for that damn hand to heal up because I was dirty from not washing properly. I will never forget that deep cut in my hand from holding onto a crack pipe too tight in my sleep.

I look back on every experience and I say, wow, man, God prepared me for all of those people that I was able to positively impact. Some of them didn't make it. But even those that didn't make it, they had a shot.

Richard: So, let me ask you this. When you came up from LA, what were your family dynamics like, what was going on in your life way back in the day? I remember how you used to tell me how you lost everything and then ended up getting everything back.

Akbar: Man, listen, I only have ten fingers, man. Actually, I didn't come directly to the Bay Area from LA. I was raised in LA, but what happened is that I was in Washington state, on my way to Alaska. But like I said, Alaska didn't work out, right. I spent a lot of time in Washington state rollin' around trying to get loaded. I remember leaving Washington on a cold, rainy night, when the wind was blowing and my clothes were wet. And you know, I just had this notion to hitchhike. A truck driver picked me up and told me he was driving down to Santa Rosa, which isn't too far from San Francisco and Oakland. The driver gave me something to eat, and we were on our way. When I finally got to San Francisco, homeless people were sleeping in the park across the street from City Hall. It was crazy, man! There were tents everywhere, and it seemed like everybody was just doing what they wanted to do. It was like paradise for me because I was using, right. I was hooked on dope, and in San Francisco I saw what I thought was drug heaven. In the morning, the police would come in and wake you up, the trash man would come in and collect all the rubbish, then people would come by and feed you breakfast, and then people would come out and donate money to all of us. I had been a responsible parent for many years, but I was thinking, "Wow! Where have I been all my life?" I didn't have to do nothing but get loaded, strangers made sure I got food, and then this guy would pass out $50 bills. I had never seen anything like that in my life, but this is what I was exposed to when I moved to San Francisco. Back then you'd have your alcoholics hangin' around in one area, and the heroin addicts would be in another area camped out, people smokin' crack over in another corner. I just made my rounds because I loved doing everything. People introduced me to the stores that you could steal from. We'd go to a store and steal a bunch of liquor, and then sell it. I got caught so many times stealing liquor, a few stores had a picture of me at the front door. I wasn't welcome in a lot of stores around town, man.

Richard: So, that was your main hustle? Boosting was your gig?

Akbar: No, that wasn't my main hustle. That was something that I did, it was just an opportunity, right. My main hustle was I would hang out at the gas station, and I would take a squeegee and I would just start cleaning car windows. I would say, "Oh my goodness, so glad I'm here. I'm going to make sure you can see clear. Because, you know, you can go to jail for impaired vision." So people just thought I was lookin' out for them, and they would give me $5, $10, sometimes they'd give me more money. All I cared about was that it kept feedin' my habit. This went on and on and on, until eventually I got so discouraged with what I saw when I looked in the mirror. I tried to avoid looking at myself as much as possible, but every now and again I would see a reflection of myself, of who I was at that time.

Man, I remember one time I was devastated and in a hopeless place about what had become of my life. I was trying to avoid feelin' sorry for myself but I couldn't help it, because, man, I was pitiful back then. I was sittin' in between two cars with some dope, but not much because it had gotten mixed in with me pickin' the crud of my feet. So I was smokin' some imaginary stuff just to get the psychological effect of having something to smoke. It was crazy, man! And while I was sittin' there, trying to maintain some semblance of being human, or decent, this man and his kid came by. I was sittin' in between two cars pickin' at my feet, one shoe on and one shoe off. I think the kid was about three or four years old, and when the kid saw me, I think I might have startled him a bit. The man grabbed his kid's hand, and they both looked at me, and then the father looked at his little son and he said to his son, "Doper!" When he said that, that kid cringed and grabbed his father's leg, and that hit me, man. That moment did something to me. I got up, and there was the Boys Club across the street on Folsom. I got up, and I went over to the Boys Club, and I looked in the mirror. And the only reason why I didn't shed any tears is because I was so dehydrated. There wasn't enough moisture in my body to cry. And in that moment when I looked at myself in the mirror, I thought, "There has to be some hope for me somewhere."

That feeling just kept getting stronger. I was suicidal at that time but I didn't want to do anything to kill myself, if that makes sense. Not only was I suicidal, but I was homicidal. A couple of guys came by one night and wanted to take what I had. I had a little wine and a little dope on me that night, and these two guys demanded that I give them what meant everything in the world to me. One thing led to another, and the next thing I know they attacked me. But they didn't know I'm straight out of Compton, right. And they didn't know that I was warding off thoughts of suicide. When they jumped on me, I went into straight self-preservation mode. There were trying to take from me the thing that had put me in my situation, and I was willing to fight to my death for it. I fought like I was fightin' for my life, fightin' for a crack pipe and a hit of dope. I got the better of them and the next thing I know, I'd gone from being the one who's being assaulted to being the assailant, right. They're hollering and yellin' for their lives and acting like I was the one that initiated the attack on them, and I'm hearing sirens, and suddenly the whole neighborhood was lit up with ambulances. I took off runnin'.

And the only place I knew as a refuge was detox. I knew Richard worked there, so that's where I went. I thought I could get Richard to hide me from everything that was going on. But of course, God always has another plan. I got down to the detox where Richard worked, and the guys working at the detox told on me. I couldn't understand that, right, because that wasn't the street code, and all the guys who told on me were from the streets. But they told the police, and the police came down to the detox.

Richard was working that night. The police asked Richard if anybody had come into his detox, and Richard said, "Yes! He's in the bathroom!" Richard told on my ass, man! I went to jail for about forty-five days fighting that case. During that time, I was able to review that whole experience, because they were talking about giving me fifteen years to life for attempted murder, and I hadn't even done anything. Those guys had jumped on me. But when one of the guys hit me with a pipe, I had taken the pipe and hit him back, and I did more damage to him than he had done to me. I had been fighting for my life. They were just trying to get what I had, so there were some different dynamics there, in a sense. That process taught me so much about being in that hopeless place and thinking that nothing was going to relieve me of that hopelessness. I called out to God in a sincere way, in a desperate way. I would pray: "I know I've said it many times before, but will you give me just one more chance. If you just give me one more chance."

The attorney who was appointed to me told me that he was able to work out a deal with the District Attorney. He could get me eleven years, and I would only do seven. My attorney was telling me, "Man, they want to get rid of you. They don't want you around the neighborhood." And I got to thinking, "Seven years? Man, I ain't doing seven years. Those guys jumped on me, man." They'd fractured my jawbone when they hit me with that pipe. But the other guy had his head cracked open from when I hit him back with the pipe.

When we were putting everything on the table, I told everyone in that room, "I'm not pleading guilty to nothin', those guys jumped on me. If I'm going to jail, it's because a jury convicts me, not because I pleaded guilty." I was angry. But I had been praying, and I had been asking God for one more chance. I started thinking, "Ok, so how am I going to organize my life to get myself together in jail? Well, I'm not going to have easy access to crack." I started visualizing myself being in the penitentiary, and I realized I felt relief: it was going to free me from that addiction. I couldn't use if I was in prison. So I said, "Ok, I'll go to prison. Whatever, I don't have any kind of life anyway." I started looking on the bright side of prison life. What else could I do?

When they called a court date, it was between the first and the third of the month, which is the time that people get their GA checks and SSI checks. One of the guys who'd jumped me was on SSI and when he got that check he took a hit of crack. He forgot he were supposed to be in court. The DA tried to get the judge to postpone the court date, but the judge said, "Hey man, these guys are supposed to be here. This guy is here incarcerated, and he's saying that they attacked him. He has a right to face his accusers, but they're not here. You have fifteen minutes to bring your guys into the courtroom or I'm dismissing the charges."

They brought me back into that holding cell for fifteen minutes, but it wasn't fifteen minutes in my mind, it was three or four months. I sat in that room agonizing, "Oh my God, please help me God." A calm came over me, and I knew that those next few minutes were in God's hands. Whatever happened was the way it was supposed to be. The bailiff came in and he said, "It looks like you are going home." And I said to him, "I don't know where that's at, but thank you very much."

When I got out of jail, my old mindset resurfaced: "Go get you a hit!" I went down on 6th Street, and right away I saw one of the guys that was trying to put me in jail. He had some dope on him, and I said, "Look man, every time I see you, you are going to give me what you got." He shared with me right away, because he knew first-hand what I was capable of, and he didn't want to go down that road with me again. The very next day I saw the other guy that tried to put me away. I was coming out of a store when we saw each other, and he ran right out in the middle of the street and he said, "Come on!" like he wanted another fight. But this other guy who I used to smoke crack with, God bless this man, because he came to me and he said, "Hey man, are you crazy? You just out of jail. They were going to give you fifteen to life. These are the guys that tried to put you away, and if you get arrested for trying to retaliate against them, man, everything is over for you." I went straight to detox after he said that. I had taken a hit of dope right when I'd gotten out of jail, when just the day before I was in jail prayin' for God to give me just one last chance. I had exhausted all those other, "give me one last chance" prayers, so I went to detox, man. And that was over twenty-seven years ago.

Richard: So, what's your clean date?

Akbar: February 16, 1997.

Richard: Tell us how you got reconnected with your family. Tell us about treatment and where you are in your life now. Because I want everyone to know that today, Mr. Akbar here is my financial mentor. I have learned so much from Akbar. Today, we do health care and wealth care, right. We help people get life insurance, 401k's, and I'm a licensed insurance agent as well. And Akbar is the marketing director for the same financial institution I work for, Global Financial Impact. I got into that because there were so many people passing away without a will or a trust, and everybody was doing GoFundMe's. People trying to retire with their little pensions, and I've been seein' people goin' back to work at seventy years old because they didn't know how money worked. They didn't understand retirement planning, and I didn't want that for my life. I started thinking about how I could get more financial stability for when I get close to retirement age, and I was introduced to this financial opportunity with Akbar. So, Akbar, tell everyone about your recovery and how you got your family back and now you're this major property owner. Man, Akbar, you are a miracle!

Akbar: When I attempted to reunite with my family, I wasn't totally aware of the trauma that my active addiction had caused a lot of the people in my life who loved and cared about me. My children had resentment toward me. My ex-wife didn't think she needed any therapy or help of any kind. When I suggested she see someone to talk about all the things that happened back in the day, my ex-wife would say, "I never smoked crack! I wasn't the one running all over the country using dope!" I remember one time I took my family to the circus and made a vow that I wasn't going to smoke any crack that night. Back then I was working a good job, making $1100 a week. And this was back in the 1980s, so that's ok money back then. With overtime, sometimes I'd bring home $1600 a week. But it never mattered, because from Friday to Monday I just couldn't seem to make it to the house with that paycheck. When I did show up, I was trying to figure out what happened to my paycheck, right. So that night, I'd promised myself I wasn't going to do some crack at the circus with my family. I hadn't used in like two weeks, and I was proud of that. But I still had my paraphernalia. I had my crack pipe in the trunk of my car, just in case. That night at the circus we watched a monkey ride on a tiger's back, and they jumped through this fiery hoop. It was amazing, man! Fireworks were going off, and it was exactly what a big circus should be. Both my kids were so happy. They were having the time of their lives. I thought, "Wow, man! This is one experience that I just want to cherish for the rest of my life." But then the nature of my disease showed up. It said, "Man, if you can just take one hit of that crack and experience this, just think how much better it would be with one hit." So I came up with a brilliant idea. I said I was going to go to the bathroom, and my son said, "I'll go with you, Daddy!" And I said, "No! I want you to watch the circus." I went out to my car and got my pipe and my crack. I got in the back seat of my car, laid down on the back floor and took a hit. To this day I don't know how my family got home from the circus.

I showed up at home that next Tuesday. I hadn't been to work. I was trying to open my front door but it wouldn't open. At first I thought my wife changed the lock on me. Turns out she was on the other side, and every time I would unlock one lock, she'd relock it. We went back and forth for a while, until finally my wife opened the door. I was like, "What's going on with the door?" She said, "Nothing is going on with the door. Where have you been?" I asked if her and the kids were ok and she said, "What does it matter to you?" After she said that, I just walked into the house, went into my room, and I laid down on my bed and tried to understand what had happened. What had compelled me to leave my family, not knowing how they would get home, and try to pretend that I was genuinely concerned. I tried to talk to the kids, but they didn't want to talk to me. Everybody in the house was a bit agitated with me. So I locked myself in my room, and I thought, "Man, I can't live like this." The dope had me thinking that the way out was not for me to stop using dope, but to just leave my family. That's how I ended up in San Francisco. I decided that I couldn't continue to abuse my family the way I had been, so I would just abandon them.

I was all caught up in crazy thinking, ideas that didn't make no damn sense. It got worse and worse over time. When I finally got into treatment in 1996, it was with all the chaos and confusion that had been the lifestyle I had lived. I didn't know how to live without lying, because what I was doing was so contrary to truth and honesty and right conduct. Telling the truth went against how I wanted to live in those dark times. When I got into a program where people cared for me, I still lied for a while. I still did things that were contrary to me getting well. I had some emotional problems and would have gotten kicked out of that program if wasn't for a few people who really supported me. I snatched a few people up a couple of times and I threatened them: "You know, if you go tell, they're going to put both of us out of this program. And if they put me out because of you telling on me, you are going to be out there with me." So they didn't tell on me. I didn't want to live like that, but I didn't know how to do anything other than what I had been doing.

Fortunately I had a counselor, Roy Washington, who was from the street. He told me, "Hey Akbar, you come meet me in my office." He took me in his office, sat me down, and he said, "Hey man, this is all off the record. You are going to get put out of this program because the staff meetings that we are having, they're always about you now. And even though I've been trying to keep you in here, man, I'm running out of alibis for you." I said to Roy, "Well, you know, man, everybody is lying about me and nobody likes me." It was always *them*. In my mind it was never my fault. I never took responsibility for me. Roy said, "Akbar you're cussing, you're yelling and being aggressive. From now on, when you get ready to say something, just put your hand over your mouth." I actually practiced doing just that. When somebody said something I didn't like, I put my hand up right over my mouth. Everybody laughed at me for a while, but it started working. I stopped saying what I wanted to say. I stopped threatening people. I stopped being profane. Things started to go so well that before I left that program, people had started calling me *Mr. Akbar*. At first this didn't mean anything to me, but after a while I started realizing that I was changing. I was changing in a good way for the first time in my life.

One day Roy brought me into his office again, but this time he told me that the conversations about me were changing. "Akbar, you are starting to do really well in this program. The conversations about you are different in staff meetings!" I was proud of myself for that, and I started priding myself into getting better every day. I shifted my mindset to get better every single day, so that's what I worked at.

Leaving that program and reuniting with my family was a whole other set of challenges. I started working during the last month that I was in my recovery program, at a job that was right up the street. I talked to Roy the first morning I was headed to work. I said, "Hey, you know, they called me to do this job just two blocks up. I can get that job done and be back in time to go over to my new program at Covenant House."

This was our original plan, right. One day after work, I called Roy to let him know I was on my way back from work so he could take me to the Covenant House program at 1:30pm. Roy replied, "Well brother, you can take your time getting back. We have to go to staff meeting and we won't be taking you to Covenant House." I said, "Why not? How am I going to get over there?" Roy said, "Well, you're not going." I panicked and felt completely abandoned in that moment. When Roy told me I wasn't going to Covenant House, I ran back down the street so I could catch Roy, and I said, "Hey man, what happened?" He explained, "Hey, man, Akbar, you know, you have done tremendous work on yourself. You are a grown man, and you are able to take care of your business. You have proven that. You don't need a secondary program. Go and get your life together, brother!" Man, I just didn't know what that meant. I was a little angry at first, and I thought for a minute, "You know, I have about $600, and I can go get me a couple of sacks and make this right in my mind." But then I said to myself, "Man, what the hell kind of crazy thinking is that?" I had been in treatment for six months, so I dismissed that thought, and I said, "Let me go and see my family."

A staff member named Herb was the only staff that took time find out where I was at and what I was doing. I still have an amazing relationship with Herb. He asked me what I was going to do, and I said, "Hey, they put me out of the program. I got clothes, but I don't know what to do with the clothes." Herb said, "Just take what you can carry." I put the items that I wanted in my suitcase, and the rest of it I donated back to the house. When he asked, "What can I do for you?" I answered, "Well, if you take me to the bus stop, I can go and see my family and see how that's going to work out." I had a few hundred on me, so I got on the Greyhound bus and I went over to Las Vegas, trying to reunite with my family. I tried to lay out a plan for my wife (now ex-wife) about how we were going to get our family back together, if that's what she wanted to do. She was happy. I spent a couple of nights out there with them. But then the place I wanted to work for, back in San Francisco, called me while I was in Las Vegas. I had to leave Las Vegas to start on that job, and the rest is pretty much history.

I kept doing what was required of me to get better every day, and every day I got better. Now, twenty-seven years later, I've got a life that I couldn't imagine would be possible for me. I have a license as a financial professional, helping people try to transition from health care to wealth care. Even though they teach you some finances when you get into college, they don't teach you the main rules of how money works. The piece that's missing from the educational process is the financial element, you see. The system is set up in such a way that all the money that working people earn, that money is actually working for somebody else. It starts off with college tuition, credit cards, loans from the bank, you know, whatever it might be. Most people, when they come out of high school or college, they got a student loan debt, they got credit card debt, and they probably got a car loan of some kind. At age thirty, they want to purchase a home, so they get another loan now. People out there have four, sometimes five debts, and they have a job that they are tied to that is responsible for them being able to pay those bills. Today we call it being a slave to your job. I was a slave to my job for over two decades. For half of my forty-three years earning money, my money had been working for somebody else. When it was time for me to retire, I had less than $100,000 in my retirement account. Now, doing this work, I realize that most working people can't retire.

I worked with a woman who had been a manager at a Walmart for thirty-two years, and when I initially started talking to her, she thought it wasn't necessary for her to worry about anything. When we looked at all of her finances, she had a $117,000. She didn't know that she had lost money in 2001, 2002, 2003, 2008, 2009. She had been losing money without even knowing. So, we educate people on how to make their money work for them instead of making somebody rich they never even met.

I could keep going on and on, telling you stories about all the people I help and how amazing my life is. But I always hesitate when I get to this portion of my story. When people ask me how my life is going, I always say, "I'm doing great! If I tell you anything else, you'll think I'm showing off." That's the kind of life that I have today.

Richard: During my journey, me and Akbar had this vision of being homeowners, and a few of us thought that we would get together and buy some property. Akbar and I got together with a couple of good friends started looking for properties in the Bay Area. At that time, my credit was in bad shape. I had started gambling, and I made some mistakes financially. But I had this girlfriend who was an accountant. She helped me clean up my credit a couple times, but I kept messing it up again. I learned how to write these dispute letters and eventually how to clean up my credit permanently, and I learned how to apply for stuff that would help me financially. I introduced her to Akbar and our other friends, they cleaned up their credit, and eventually it was time to come up with the money. Everybody was supposed to come up with $7000. At the time I didn't have that kind of money because of the gambling, so I couldn't be a part of the first investment that I helped set up. Akbar and our two other friends ended up buying that first property, but I had the money needed for the next investment. On that first investment, I knew I could still help renovate the property and invest in that way. Akbar ended up buying out the other investors, so he owned the whole property, which had cost about $300,000. Today that four-bedroom fourplex in Oakland's Maxwell Park neighborhood is worth four times what it was originally bought for.

I remember one time my car was towed from Turk and Fillmore, so my wife and I were stuck. I called Akbar, and he paid to get my car back, picked me and my wife up, and let me know I needed to stop gambling. I stopped going to casinos, and for the last two or three years I haven't done any kind of gambling. It just isn't worth it.

Akbar is the reason I have the job I have now. I lost my job at Haight Ashbury Free Clinics when Walden House and Haight Ashbury Free Clinics merged. I settled for a case manager job over at Center Point, and I worked that job for three years. Every time I would try to get a promotion, they would deny me. Akbar was the one that told me, "Man, you are settling for mediocrity! You used to be a boss. You are better than what you are doing. You have been doing this way too long, you're smarter than half of the supervisors there. Why are you still there?" When Akbar said this to me, I knew I was done with Center Point. I applied for a manager's job where I work now, with Tenderloin Housing Clinic. Because of my experience, they gave me the job making way more money than I was making at Center Point. I have been promoted four times, and today I'm the only black director on the THC executive team We have four hundred employees, and I have a good relationship with the founder of THC, Randy Shaw. It's all because Akbar motivated me when he said things like, "Man, the worst thing with black people or anybody with low self-esteem and low self-worth is that they settle for mediocrity." Akbar reminded me that I was a boss, a supervisor, that I am intelligent, I have skills, and I could do so much more with my life.

Our relationship started when we were out there using, then we came into recovery. We've been best friends, supporting each other in our recovery, me and 6th Street Sid. I always joke, I know his plantation name, Sydney Smith. I'm probably one of the only people that knows this information. I know his family; I was able to help his brother. His kids look at me like Uncle Richard B., and Akbar and I, we are family. Akbar and I have been brothers for three decades, from 6th Street Sid, to stealing his pipe, to now being homeowners and property owners. I encouraged him to get clean back when I worked at the detox, and then he encouraged me by telling me that I could do better in my life. So, I just want to say to you Akbar, that you are my best friend and I'll love you til the end. 6th Street Sid a.k.a. Salahudin Akbar.

Akbar: No, no, it's Salahudin Akbar a.k.a. 6th Street Sid.

Richard: Hey, before we close up, is there anything else you want to say to the person that is reading this right now?

Akbar: Don't stop, wherever you are. I think it was Arthur Ash who said, *Start where you are*. Stevie Wonder said, *Destination is the brightest star*. And then Les Brown came back with, *Is it better to aim high and miss, or to aim low and hit your bulls-eye?* We all got choices. I'm going to keep aiming high, even though I might miss. You might miss the moon, but you'll land amongst the stars. And so there it is, brother. Everybody got their own challenges in life. You know, we all start where we are. But if we don't ever get started, we'll just stay where we are.

CHAPTER 5

Teflon-Coated Recovery

I know I've mentioned some of this before but I really want to make it clear how tough you have to be to get clean and stay clean in the Tenderloin. You got to have Teflon-coated recovery. A friend of mine used to say, *recovery is a hero's journey, suckers don't make it*. I never wanted to be a sucker. I'm a baller. I'm this, I'm that. But I ain't no sucker. And my friend told me I was a sucker to the disease of addiction. I really heard this. What he said really stuck with me. At first, I didn't know what he meant by *the disease of addiction*. I had never heard that before. I didn't know anything about the disease of addiction. I would learn that the disease of addiction tricks you all the time. It tells you to do things you don't want to do, and go places you don't want to go. It takes away your appetite, you can't eat, all your money gets spent on dope. That's the disease of addiction, man. When I decided to stop running around and acting like a fool, I had all these resources all around me. I didn't want to go back to Richmond, so I decided to stay right here in San Francisco and get clean for good. So I went into the program. And that first week or two in the program, I didn't like it. I didn't like being in the dining room, I didn't like people telling me what to do all the time. I didn't like sleeping in a room with other men. I did like the structure of the program, and the people that showed me some love and genuine concern. There was this guy, Melvin Harris, who was my first sponsor. But he relapsed. A guy named Don was a counselor at the program as well. Don went to jail. He was doing stuff that was not conducive to his recovery, and he ended up in jail clean. Two or three other counselors there died. This is all since I have been clean over the past twenty-nine years and two months and so many days. I saw all of that, man, but during my first thirty days at St. Anthony's, man, I made the decision to give recovery a chance.

One dude told me, "You ain't got to use, even if you want to." He told me not to go to any stores that sell alcohol, because people hang around those stores where alcohol is sold. They'll wait right outside and offer you some rock right when you're trying to leave the store. He told me to identify the stores in my area that don't sell any alcohol and go just to those stores. That piece of simple advice saved my life, man. I was told to keep my hands in my pockets when I walked around all the stores in the Tenderloin. Just keep walking and keep your hands in your pockets. Whenever I asked why, everyone would tell me because if I don't pick up, I won't get loaded. This was all new to me back then, man. I used those little tools that were being given to me. For a while my mind would tell me to go in those stores and get a beer, but I had that tool that I learned: just keep your hands in your pockets, keep walking, and you'll be alright. So that's what I did.

Over time I gathered more tools from people who wanted to see me succeed. I would put those tools in my toolbox, and I would move on to the next step. I'd never heard of a toolbox before, but here I was with a toolbox full of tools that were keeping me alive, right. And I used all those tools while walking in the Tenderloin. In the Tenderloin, every block has a liquor store with a bunch of guys waiting for you to come out with your beer so they can offer you some dope. There is a whole system in the TL designed to keep you down, so you got to have some tools in order to survive. Only one or two stores in the Tenderloin didn't sell alcohol, but I knew exactly where they were, and that's where I went. As a matter of fact, the first people I really learned how to develop relationships with were the people that worked at those stores that didn't sell alcohol. The guys that worked there knew me, the owners knew me, the owners' friends and family knew me. This is how I got my start. I also never went into bars or clubs in those early days. There's no way I would have made it if I went into those places. There's just no way. These tools allowed me to develop my Teflon-coated recovery.

I used to read about John Gotti. Everybody was tryin' to bring him down, and I remember seeing him on all these magazine covers calling him "The Teflon Don." I said, "I gotta have 'Teflon-coated recovery.'" My recovery had to stand all the tests that would come my way. It didn't matter if my brother came by or my mother came by, because some people in our lives are triggers for us. In our groups, we would talk about people who are triggers. The way they say things, the way they talk, the way they walk. "Hey man, let's go hit this store, let's go to this alley, let's go to this place over here." I realized that some people would remind me of things I used to do. Some people would look like a straight-up crack pipe to me with the things they would say to me, and some people would look like a 40oz. All we'd done was drink together, so that's what they reminded me of. There are these women that all you did was tweak and then freak with them. I had to stay away from all that, man. I can't hang with those women, I can't hang with Mr. 40oz. I gotta be tough. I gotta get through all of this stuff. I can't be the one that fails this time. I can't be the one that gets tore up this time. I can't be the one where the counselor says, "Look around at everyone in this group. There are about fifty people in here, right? Only one or two of you are going to make it." I told myself, *I'm going to be one of those two.*

When I worked in the dining room at St. Anthony's, in the Tenderloin, triggers were all around me. I was what you called "the runner." The runner had to take the garbage from the dining room and take it over to the parking lot, down Golden Gate Avenue and then over to Leavenworth Street. I'd dump the garbage and come back, which meant I was out on the street all the time, seein' people on the sidewalk smoking dope. The drug dealers own Leavenworth, so I'm bobbin' and weavin' through all of this, pushing a garbage can with an apron on that says St. Anthony's Dining Room. All these dope dealers I'm seeing, they remembered me. They knew who I was. They knew that I was the one that used to be out there on the streets all tore up, hangin' out and buying dope. I started out a slinger and ended up a carpet cleaner and a blinds inspector. You know, someone that picks through their carpet for hours, looking for little crumbs of dope in the floor and constantly lookin' out their window in case the man is looking for them. I was all of those things, man. Everybody knew what I used to be. But they also knew that I was in a program. Everybody knew about St. Anthony's and Glide. I owed some of those dope dealers a little money, but they always used to tell me that as long as I was clean I didn't owe them any money. As soon as I relapsed, I'd owe that money again. I never relapsed, man! Some of those guys are still waiting for their money, almost thirty years later, man. Back then, in my early sobriety days, I was just so set on not using. I tried just smoking weed. Didn't work. I tried just drinking. It didn't work. I always ended up going back to crack. So finally I decided it was total abstinence from now on. I was determined to be that one guy out of fifty who was going to be clean and stay clean.

My roommate from those early days of recovery was named "Gator." We went to a lot of places together, challenging each other on things like who had on the best tennis shoes. We would check on each other constantly in order to make sure the other one didn't relapse. Gator is still clean today as well. In October 2024, he celebrated twenty-nine years. Our clean dates are like three months apart from each other. But early in our recovery, Gator would deviate every night. He would go out with these guys who would say they were going to an NA meeting or an AA meeting, but they would go to their girlfriend's house instead or go to the movies with old friends who were still using. I told Gator, "Look man, if you want to go out and do that stuff, you do you, but don't ask me to do that with you, man. As a matter of fact, if you keep running around with those guys, you *will* relapse. So, I need you to keep that stuff away from me, man. What you are doing isn't conducive to your sobriety and I ain't messin' with any of that." I knew that none of those guys cared about my recovery. The girls they were hangin' with didn't care about anything but gettin' high, so I stayed as far away from them as possible. I wasn't going to relapse, and I wasn't going to be a sucker to no girl. Bein' around the kind of men that I was raised up with, the first thing I learned was, don't trust a woman that's into drugs and that fast life. It's that simple, man. When I was coming up in the game, every man that I ever saw go down, a woman was involved. Plus, I had issues of my mother abandoning me as a kid, so I didn't trust women. Every one of those guys that was deviating from their recovery, every one of them relapsed behind a woman, and vice versa. Every one of them. That's a true story. My first sponsor always told me that most people relapse because of romance or finances. Luckily, Gator eventually started to listen to me.

When recovery started working for me, showing some positives in my life, making me feel like I had some self-esteem and some self-worth again, I started remembering some of the things my grandmother and father taught me about standing up and being a man. A man is a provider, a man is always supposed to be strong, but dope and bad decisions make a man weak. I had to accept that a lot of my decisions were making me a weak man. Having the disease of addiction doesn't make me weak. It's the decisions that I make that make me a strong man or a weak man.

I remember I tried telling my father that he shouldn't be smoking pot around my little brothers. My father said to me, "Hold on, I'll be right back." He came back downstairs with his pistol in his hand, and he said, "Man, don't you ever tell me what to do in my house, boy!" I just looked at him and said, "Yes sir." My father taught me a lesson on that day. I can't tell anybody what to do, especially my own father, man. I can't tell people what to do just because I got clean. I can't tell people how to live their life.

This is what I mean by Teflon-coated recovery. I couldn't let anybody knock me off my square, no matter how close they were to me. The symbol of Narcotics Anonymous is a square inside a circle. The circle represents a universal program—everybody is in the circle. But not everybody is in the square. I had to realize that a lot of people who claim to be in recovery or are trying to get into recovery are not practicing the spiritual principles. I found that with people who were still sellin' dope in recovery or still hustling in recovery.

I had an opportunity to be a methadone counselor, but I turned it down because I truly believe that people on methadone are still addicted to a drug. It treats the symptom, but not the disease of addiction. It takes the edge off the withdrawal, but it doesn't treat the disease. Knowing that, I decided that I wanted to be a role model for my family members who were struggling with addiction, and I wanted to be a role model for my friends and for my community. My little brother, who was only eight years old when our father passed away, he had needed a positive role model. That same baby brother just got sentenced to life in prison for first-degree murder. He got into it over a girl. He chased a guy into an apartment complex, and my brother put him on his knees and shot that man in the back of his head. My baby brother executed that man over a woman. They call that *great bodily harm* because he shot him in the back of the head. And when you get someone on their knees, that's premeditated. My brother never confessed; he always said he didn't do it, but the evidence says otherwise. Dark times, man. But in recovery, things don't have to be like that. Life can be good. We need role models to show us how good life can be.

While heavy things were happening to people I loved, like my brothers and some of my old friends from back in the day, all I could think about was building up the foundation of my recovery. The recovery community and the range of programs and services in San Francisco were incredible. I met Bob Berg (he gave me my first coffee commitment), and another guy named Frank Brennon. Frank had over fifty years clean. He was big into AA, and he stayed at the Arlington Hotel over on Ellis and Leavenworth. The Arlington, run by the John Stewart Property Management Group, was the first model of a clean and sober transitional housing building in San Francisco, and for years it was the only one. A lot of people who completed treatment would try to get into the Arlington. Everybody in the recovery sphere knew and loved

Frank. And then, of course you had Glide. Glide had so many programs, like the Men in Motion, Women on the Move, Facts on Crack, and the Circle Program.

San Francisco, back in the '90s, was the gold standard of recovery. People would come from all over the world to get clean in San Francisco. Today, people are coming from all over to get loaded. They are coming from all over to get dope now. In the '90s there were faith-based programs, Salvation Army, outpatient programs at Glide, Walden House, and Haight Ashbury Free Clinic. Dr. David Smith was the father of addiction medicine for San Francisco. He was the man. He wrote numerous books on addiction. And then there was Dr. Darryl Inaba, who wrote *Uppers, Downers, All Arounders*, part of the curriculum to get certified as an alcohol and drug counselor. I thought I was the man because I was going to school to become an alcohol and drug counselor and I had direct access to the guy that wrote the book. Dr. Inaba was the director and program director for the Haight Ashbury Free Clinic, and Dr. Greg Hanner was an important pharmacist.

Back then all these programs and people were working together. This is when the medical model and the mental health model started to integrate and developed into behavioral health. Substance abuse, mental health, and behavior started getting looked at holistically instead of as separate issues. Also in the '90s, Prop 36 was passed, so that people were getting mandated into treatment. The first treatment on demand program was at 1380 Howard Street. Part of the new behavioral health model included offering needle exchange; in San Francisco various Ryan White programs were trying to impact the AIDS epidemic. I ended up running Western Addition Recovery House, where the target population was HIV positive African American males. It was the only program in the city that targeted that population. Many people there were struggling with both the virus and addiction. In addition to the needle exchange program, we gave out condoms. This was the early harm reduction movement, before providers started giving out free pipes or anything like that. The only things we were giving out were condoms and clean needles in order to slow the spread of the HIV virus. At one point it was illegal to do needle exchange, but people were doing it anyway. San Francisco could do it, but most cities didn't allow it.

San Francisco was the starting place for so many movements. We were the first to have free medical services based on the philosophy that "health is a right, not a privilege." And remember, it was Haight Ashbury *Free* Clinic. There were no free clinics before San Francisco did it. We were trailblazers out here, man! We were serious about doing addiction medicine back in the beginning. I mean, we had conventions coming out here, both AA and NA. I would go to a convention with thousands of people in Union Square, all of them clean, and recovery was strong. It wasn't like the UN Plaza is today, with an open-air drug market. When I got clean in the late '90s, things were amazing. But after 2010, a lot of things changed. The court system wanted to shift away from 12-step recovery and toward something that could actually be measured; since 12-step programs are anonymous, you can't get real data to prove how effective 12-step recovery really is. When I was in treatment, you had to complete each step before you could go to the next phase of your recovery. This kept us each moving forward and always progressing. To me and many others, this is definite proof that the 12-step model is effective.

Twelve-step recovery was the basis for the social model programs. Behavior modification was the basis for the attack therapy kind of programs. Faith-based programs were based on God and Jesus and all that. Those were the three big modalities, or programs, back then, and they were all very strong. AA, NA, even Cocaine Anonymous was coming up; meetings were offered all over the city. We had 99th Street, the Dry Dock, all the churches, The Gratitude Center, you name it man, you couldn't walk two blocks without knowing that you could go to a meeting. It was overwhelming, man, but in a good way. You could go to two or three different meetings back-to-back on the same block in the Tenderloin back then. It was wild! I did two or three meetings a day for my first five years of recovery. Post and Mason Street, three hundred people every Monday, Friday, and Saturday. That was the biggest meeting in the city, and it was dress to impress.

I was the coffee maker for those meetings at Post and Mason. Bob Burr was the treasurer of that meeting, and he used to keep a little 22 pistol in his jacket pocket because people tried to rob him after the meeting a few times. My side hustle back then was I used to sell body oil right outside the meetings to make some extra cash. I would be outside the meeting selling my body oil, and Bob Burr would tell me, "Hey man, you can't sell that body oil out here, man!" And I'd say, "Hey man, this is an outside issue. Mind your business, old man." One day Bob said, "Hey, you need to be here early tomorrow. I want to show you something." So I came to the next meeting early. I met up with Bob, and he walked me over to the coffee pot and he said, "I now pronounce you man and wife. You may kiss the bride!" Bob married me to the coffee maker. He told me I was going to make coffee from now on. I never asked for how long, and Bob never told me how long. Bob was funny as hell, man. Back in the day, people gave you commitments. Nobody was asking you for permission back then. If an old timer told you to show up for something, you didn't question it. You just showed up. It's different now. If you have been in recovery a while, you know a lot of things are different today. Back then we had the A-B-C's: ashtrays, brooms, and chairs. You see, back then, people were still smoking in the meetings. You would come and set up the meeting, sweep the floors, dump the ashtrays, you know, the A-B-C's. After I was assigned to be the coffee maker, I made the best coffee, man. I was proud of my strong coffee. I'd stand by the coffee machine and would ask everyone, "Would you like some coffee? Would you like some sugar with your coffee? Cream?" I just loved it when the girls would give me a hug, "Oh, Richard B., that coffee sure was good. Let's give it up for the coffee maker, Richard B.!" That would get three hundred people clapping for me, and who wouldn't want to come back for that, right? Those were some exciting times back then, man. Being the coffee maker really built up my self-esteem. It made me want to come back for more. I never had that feeling when I was using and hustling, man.

I was always told that people who do service stay clean. No matter how much time you have, if you do service, you will stay clean. So I kept doing service, man, and I still do service to this day. I've been secretary for the Men's Breakfast Committee for the Peninsula for the last fifteen years. I always believe in doing service and sponsoring people and maintaining a positive atmosphere for recovery.

Back then I was going to AA, NA, any A that would save my ass, right. I went to all of them. Saint Mary's Cathedral had the big AA meetings, and the big NA meeting was that one on Post and Mason Street. I would go there on chip night, and I would get my chip on. "Oh, man, it's chip night tonight, baby!" Me and my boys would all be dressed to the nines, and I'd go up and get my ninety-day chip! I loved dressing up for chip night, man. Then you'd get your six-month chip, and then would come that big one-year chip, man. I still have my one-year chip.

For years, some of the wrong girls would try to get at me, and some of the guys would try to get me to do stuff that wasn't good for my recovery, but I just deflected all of that stuff. That's why we call it Teflon-coated recovery, man! I listened to my sponsor and I did what he did. After eight years, my sponsor relapsed. That really taught me something, because he relapsed behind a relationship. All I could think to myself was, "Man, how are you going to go out over some woman, man? Now I have to get myself another sponsor." Then I got another sponsor named Jessie, who was the founder of the Men in Motion Program over at Glide. Men in Motion eventually moved over to the art theater gallery on 6th and Market. We rented that gallery for our meetings there on Wednesdays at 7:00. I was the secretary for that meeting and for the business meeting for eight years. We would do Men in Motion dances, and then we started Recovery Day at Boeddeker Park. For the first Recovery Days, we would go to the park with a microphone and just talk. We would tell stories about recovery, and let people know that there was a better way to live if you were struggling with addiction. Recovery Day is off the chain today.

We have great food, music, and vendors and community groups bringing information about new recovery programs. We started doing Recovery Day in the '90s, but it stopped in 2000. I brought it back in 2020, and it's better than ever.

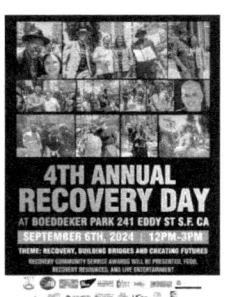

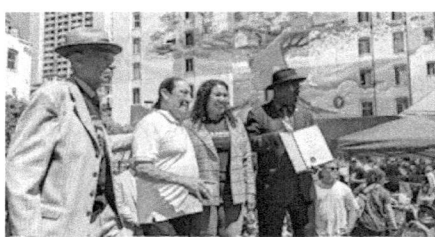

Del from the TL, Danny Trejo, Mayor London Breed, and me receiving a Certificate of Honor at Recovery Day

And you know, my Men in Motion brothers, we were all tight. We would go on "Street Soldiers" on the radio with Dr. Joe Marshall, and we would speak about all the things that were going on in San Francisco. We would go to Omega Boys Club to talk to all the kids. We would go inside the jails, we would go inside all the different institutions. We would take turns speaking at each place we went to. Men in Motion helped build my recovery foundation 100%, man. There was some real recovery goin' on, man. Teflon-coated recovery.

Things changed. I think the two major things that led to this change were the growth of harm-reduction programs, and covid. Covid shut down everything, and then the county health-care administrators said that 12-step programs were not evidence based. They said there was no data to prove that it was effective treatment. So a lot of people no longer saw going to 12-step meetings as going to treatment, and the courts stopped mandating people to go to 12-step meetings. For years judges had told people to go to AA meetings, but the courts have backed away from that. Around the same time, faith-based programs lost their government funding because they didn't practice harm-reduction principles. The whole atmosphere of recovery changed: 12-step programs lost their credibility as evidence-based treatment and the system stopped sending people to meetings. Instead they sent you to therapy; the system says everybody needs therapy and SSRIs now. I'm not saying that therapy doesn't work. I'm not against therapy. But back in the day, either you were clean or you weren't. Today the system has all these loopholes for people who are addicts. People are being prescribed weed, methadone, or ketamine by doctors, while 12-step programs aren't even in the back of these doctors' minds anymore. The outlook on how to treat addiction has changed.

And of course, covid really changed things. Covid shut meetings down, separated people from their kids. When covid hit, you *really* had to have Teflon-coated recovery, because all we had were those Zoom meetings. I started one of the first Zoom meetings in my area immediately when covid hit; there was no choice. It took a long period of time to get back to brick and mortar meetings and away from Zoom, but I'm actually grateful for Zoom meetings, man. I have been able to build relationships with people from all over the world. People from Australia, Canada, New Zealand, South Africa, and all over Europe. In fact, I recently spoke to an NA meeting in Kenya, thanks to Zoom. Another thing I like about Zoom meetings is that you can wake up at 4:00 in the morning and get on a Zoom meeting. If you really need a meeting, you go on Zoom and get yourself a meeting. But nothing can replace real friendship, a good hug from someone you trust, shaking hands with another sober man or woman. You can't do any of that on a screen, man. But if you are disabled, bed ridden, or hurt in some way, Zoom is really a life saver.

I still see that something is missing, and San Francisco needs to go back to being that gold standard. We need more AA and NA meetings in the city. As the Director of Recovery Services for Tenderloin Housing Clinic now, I want to bring AA and NA into every one of the twenty-three buildings that we have. I want to bring that atmosphere of recovery back into San Francisco. I push it with my team, and I voice it to the executive team of THC and with Randy Shaw, the founder of Tenderloin Housing Clinic. I think if you want to make real change in the world, first you have to be completely honest regarding what is going on. Right now, in early 2025, AA and NA meetings in San Francisco have fallen off, and I am determined to help change that. San Francisco is an amazing city with amazing people, and if we all work together, we can bring San Francisco back to that gold standard of recovery. Giving out free pipes and foil to addicts is not where we want to be. We need to go back to the old-school way, because the old-school way worked.

CHAPTER 6

The Always Powerful Kim Vicious

K im, thank you for being willing to interview for the book, *Recovering From The Game*. I wanted a female in the book, and you were the first person that came to mind. You are my sister in recovery. You are someone with a powerful story and message. You already know that I am a big cheerleader when it comes to your recovery, and I am so happy that you agreed to be in this book. So, I want to introduce all of you to Ms. Kim Vicious!

Kim: Ok, well, it all started when my mother married a man who went by Pistol Pete. Pete was my introduction into the game back in the mid '70s. The lifestyle, the fast-paced life, and the whole fascination of it. While Pistol Pete was in San Quentin, we used to write letters trying to get him out. Finally, Pete got out and within two years he was in Oakland, in the game, doing everything to make money. But my mom wasn't happy with what was going on. My mother was a nurse, and she wanted a more stable lifestyle for her and her family. I was barely a teenager, but I was all in it. I wanted to do everything I saw Pete doing. I loved all the Cadillacs and the nice clothes and all the jewelry. I wanted all of it!

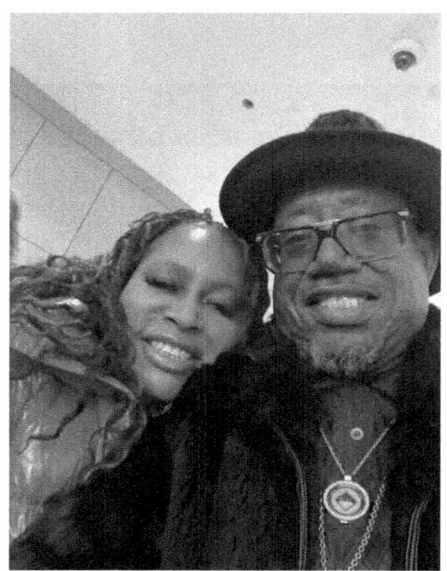

Kim V. and the Ambassador

For a while, Pistol Pete teamed up with a guy and they became inseparable, making a lot of money together. This is around the time when I got into the game and was getting loaded. My mom could see how turned on I was by everything that was going on, so she tried to keep me out of that lifestyle. She got me into modeling, which put more money into my pocket, and I would put that money back into the game I was running. Eventually started working with another individual that I met through Pete, and they taught me how to buy and sell dope, how to flip it and turn it around, how to work with other women, how to control them and make more money off them. Everything seemed to happen so fast, and I was just off and running doing my own thing. And then, the next thing you know, I had moved from being a part of the game to running the game.

After some time, I met this guy named Rico, and I ended up marrying him. Rico came from a powerful, notorious family that was deep into the game, right. They were into everything. Rico's brother, Shawn, he got robbed for a hundred grand and there was a price on the heads of the people that robbed him, but that situation was just a drop in the bucket for this family. There was always some kind of shooting happening, people getting robbed, revenge was always right around the corner and money was everywhere. I was completely fascinated by my husband and his family. If Rico said jump, I'd say how high, right. That's just kind of how that went back then. And from that point on, that was my lifestyle. You know, selling dope, boosting, shooting, stabbings, you name it. Rico was in and out of the penitentiary, and then I got pregnant. When I got pregnant, I had my first introduction into Narcotics Anonymous. I knew I needed to make some changes when I got pregnant. Right when I got into NA, I kind of got with a new guy who everybody called "Funky Rat." He used to take NA meetings into San Quentin Prison. So I was in Narcotics Anonymous with this new guy, and I was skimming the surface of NA but I wasn't really doing any of the work. I was kind of just his girl, and that was my focus then. When that relationship faded I left Narcotics Anonymous and went back out to the streets and back into the game. Then things got dark really fast. While Rico was in prison, I ended up getting stabbed thirteen times while six months pregnant with my son. The man that stabbed me is still in prison to this day, doing twenty-five years to life. My son is now thirty years old, and we both made it out of the hell I was living all those years.

Richard: Can you talk more about the stabbing situation that you just mentioned? The stabbing is a big part of your story, and I think we should get into it.

Kim: Ok, well, the story is blurred and the complete truth never came out, so we never got the clarity we needed to understand why the stabbing happened. When my husband Rico went to jail, I was trying to keep our business going. The man that would end up stabbing me was originally doing some business with us on occasion. My husband's family didn't really like me, because I stole him away from another chick who Rico's family really liked. The man that stabbed me was really close with Rico's family, and the stabbing was a hit on me, because I was pregnant with Rico's child and Rico's family didn't want me to have the baby. So, this guy came by a few times to buy product from me, and one night he just pushed his way through as I was opening the door. He grabbed me by my neck and ended up stabbing me thirteen times in the neck. Everything happened so fast that at first I didn't realize I was being stabbed. My adrenaline was that high! Originally, I thought he was trying to rape me. I was on the floor gasping for air, and I noticed blood was all over the floor, and that's when I realized this guy was trying to kill me. I stopped fighting him, closed my eyes, and pretended that I was dead. I just laid still. He got off me and started ransacking the house, took all the product and the money that I had in the house, washed his hands in the bathroom, and left. When I tried to get up, I realized that I couldn't move my head. I rolled over to the phone and there was even more blood on the floor and all over my hands. I was able to call 911, and I was taken to the hospital. I can remember being in the ambulance and everyone in the ambulance kept saying, "She's not going to make it, she's not going to make it!" I told them to do whatever they had to do to save my baby. But of course, as you can see today, we both made it. Right after all that happened, I had to go to two trials. Since I had a criminal record they were trying to make it seem like I was involved in a deal that went bad, and I asked for all this trouble that went down, right. They offered the guy that stabbed me twelve years, but he wouldn't take it. They took him to trial a second time, and he ended up getting twenty-five-years-to-life in prison. He was the first man convicted of the three-strikes-you're-out law in San Mateo County. When covid hit, he tried to get a covid release. The attorneys called me and asked me if I wanted to add in the report why I wanted him to stay in prison, but I just stayed out of all that. I let the courts know that I didn't have anything to say for or against him.

That was all a turning point for me, because I think I became a bit more psychotic after that stabbing incident. You know, going through that kind of violence changed me. It became hard for me to do things that I used to be able to do. Holding down a job became impossible for me. Even though I was hustling, I was also gainfully employed, but it became too difficult for me to be out in the world for a long time. I went deeper into illegal activities, and I started using and drinking more. I went off the deep end for a while, and it was a long road trying to get back. I even ended up in prison myself. I went to prison for two years for armed robbery and for possession for sales. My walk in prison is what really brought me to the program of Narcotics Anonymous, but for real this time. I wasn't playin' around anymore. I never would have thought that a series of tragedies like the ones I just described to you would bring me to my true self. I was in prison with people who were lifers, baby killers, real deal murderers. It was incredible and overwhelming. Prison was like no other experience I had ever had before. I went to Valley State Prison for Women in 2009 and I got out at the end of 2010. When I got out, I immediately went into a recovery program, which started a journey of changing my life around. I didn't know how I was going to do it, so I just did what everybody told me to do. I ended up getting a sponsor and getting a job through the program. I started working with other women and eventually I came back to the Bay Area. That's when I met Richard Beal. Richard and I spoke at a recovery convention in the Bay Area. Soon after we spoke at the convention, Richard turned me onto a new job working in the recovery field, where I would be able to help people dealing with addiction issues. Over the years I have been able to climb the ladder with work, but things haven't been easy all the way. There have been some situations in my life that haven't been great, like I got involved with another man that was in prison. I kind of ran with him for about seven years while I was in sobriety, so I know I still have this fascination with the lifestyle. I have always had this fascination with the game and the fast-paced life. Even though I have fifteen years clean, there is a certain type of individual that I like hanging out with. I still hang around the pimps, the hustlers, and the players of the world, and that's just who I am, right. There might never be anything I can do to change that. But I have changed my ways and my attitude and ideas, and I do things differently today.

Richard: Tell us about your sponsees and all the work that you do in NA.

Kim: Oh, yeah, now we're talking about something that I really want to go into. My clean date is 4/15/09. And since I've been clean, I've worked with a bunch of women in NA. I had one sponsee that committed suicide. When I'd moved back out to the Bay Area, I'd immediately started with this one woman. One night we were talking on the phone and I could tell something was wrong, so I told her I was going to stop by her place so we could talk more in person. But before I could get to her, she had already passed away. Another woman that I sponsored had been to the penitentiary too. We became really close, and we have been working together for nine years now. I met my second sponsee in a NA meeting, and there was some kind of kindred attraction between us. We have been working together for almost ten years as well. Another one of my sponsees, she had about five years clean when I met her, and she ended up relapsing while we were working together. This was devastating for both of us. I felt like it reflected on me as a sponsor, like it was kind of my fault that she relapsed, right. I remember telling her, "Hey, if you want to get another sponsor, that's totally fine with me. I understand. Whatever it takes for you to stay clean, you do that." I really wanted her to get this program, and I didn't want to stand in the way of that. But she told me, "Kim, look, I don't want to work with anybody else. I just want to work with you. My relapse had nothing to do with you. That was all me." She has since worked her way back to having five more years clean, and she's working on six. We've been on quite a journey together, and right now we are in Los Angeles together, both sharing at a Narcotics Anonymous Convention. The relationship that we have is almost stronger than a relationship between two sisters. There is nothing that I don't know about her and there's nothing that she doesn't know about me. To watch people grow like this, this is why I'm here. This is why I stay clean.

I have lost some sponsees along the way, but I know God puts people in your life for a reason and that's ok. It's all good, right. At the end of the day, it's all about the work that we do, because I can only keep what I have by giving it away. So that's what I do today. Today, I probably

RECOVERING FROM THE GAME – 84

have ten sponsees, maybe six of them do the work. When I say *do the work*, I mean we have gone through the 12 steps of Narcotics Anonymous and we start seeing who we are and sorting through all the contradictions and confusion that goes on inside of our heads. We talk about being a servant of the spirit. We dig deep down inside of who we are, and we find out what it is that makes us want to get loaded and live that dark lifestyle. The 12 steps are a game changer. When you get to Narcotics Anonymous, your whole life ends up changing. You don't have to change everything all at once, but you have to change at least one thing in the beginning: your belief system and the way that you think. It's not necessarily a drug problem that we have, it's a living problem that we have. The way that we deal with situations and different people in society on an everyday basis, that's the real problem.

I feel like I gain more every day. I've had one sponsee since she was twenty-two years old. She's thirty years old now, clean, in this program, having relationships, making mistakes, going through life sober. I have made it my life's work to help women and try to teach them and show them that they are valuable, that they are worthy members of Narcotics Anonymous. I want to show them that the sky is the limit. I want to help these women step into their greatness. Because there's a greatness that comes with having these two lives that I've had. I had that life in the game, and now I have this new life where I live in the light. This life in recovery, helping other women find their light.

Richard: You remember my sponsee, Bruce, right? I know you were close with Bruce back in the day. Can you take a minute to talk about your friendship with Bruce? You and Bruce were like brother and sister, and you don't see that every day in recovery.

Kim: Yes, so Bruce was a gentleman who came from the East Coast, and he just couldn't get this program. But the thing about Bruce is he had this hope and this beautiful big heart, he literally brought the NA fellowship in San Francisco together. Many people were divided and would not talk to each other, but everybody loved Bruce. I met Bruce when I first started working at the place I'm at now. Bruce lived right around the corner from the site I worked at, so I would go by his place and check on him. I would stop by and talk with him, I would make sure that he was eating, and I'd take him to meetings, so Bruce would get bouts of clean time. But in the end, Bruce just could not get this program of Narcotics Anonymous. Bruce wouldn't do the rigorous work that needed to be done for him to stay clean. I ended up getting a promotion and moved over to another site, and my new work site wasn't around the corner from Bruce anymore. I heard that he was going to meetings, but I lost touch with him for a while. One day I ran into Bruce and he told me he had less than a day sober, so I swooped him up and I took him to a meeting out in Modesto, which is like a two-hour drive. Bruce was so angry with me, because he was stuck in the car with me and he couldn't go anywhere. His disease of addiction was calling him, and he couldn't go anywhere. When I finished sharing at the meeting in Modesto, Bruce raised his hand and he said, "I have three hours clean!" It was so powerful. The room just erupted. It was one of those "Welcome to Narcotics Anonymous" moments. After that meeting, I knew he was going to meetings sporadically, but people would tell me that Bruce just kept getting loaded. A lot of the NA community was starting to get angry with Bruce, because they were putting so much time into helping him but he kept disappearing and using. After a couple of months, I went by Bruce's place in an SRO. I told the front desk person that I'd found a better place for Bruce, and the SRO employee needed to open Bruce's door for me so I could talk to him. When they opened up the door, there he was. Bruce was sunk over his bed; he had a crack pipe in one hand and a pen in his other hand. Bruce was lying on top of his Narcotics Anonymous Step Work Guidebook. Bruce was gone. This was the day that I learned that some people can have the desire to stay clean but for whatever reason, they just can't stay clean. Bruce is a chapter all on its own. And I'll tell you this. I have never seen a person, a newcomer, with so many people in the program of Narcotics Anonymous that showed up for their funeral. There so many people at Bruce's funeral. It was amazing! The fellowship buried Bruce. Bruce didn't have family.

Richard: Yeah, Bruce had an infectious personality. He was funny, he was kind, and he was real. But he couldn't stay clean. I loved Bruce. But I want to say this, Kim. You know how some people will see something special in you but you might not see it in yourself? I feel that I saw some things in you, back when you were in early recovery, that you might not have seen yourself. I think you see it now, but I don't think you saw just how powerful your message was in the beginning. I don't think you realized how much power you had. And then we ended up going to Pittsburgh.

Kim: Oh, yeah, that was huge.

Richard: You and I shared a hotel room together, as brother and sister, strictly platonic, because we are like family. We were in Pittsburgh for an NA Convention and my sponsor was one of the main speakers. I did a workshop and Kim did a workshop. And that was the first time Kim had traveled three thousand miles to be of service on that level, and Kim shared her ass off.

Kim: Yeah, that was a big moment in my life. On the East Coast, they had been doing Narcotics Anonymous a little bit longer than the West Coast had been doing it, so there were people that had a lot more time than me. I had four years clean back then. Some of the people were challenging me, asking me if I was speaking at the convention. It was a little intimidating for me at the time. But when you stand up and talk about something that you believe in, it's not *on* you, it's *in* you, and everything seemed to come naturally to me.

I want to add that Richard has been instrumental in my life. As I have grown in the program, I haven't needed him as much as I did in the beginning. Richard taught me how to not need him. Richard is the type of person who sees something in a person and knows how to cultivate it and pull it out of you. Richard knows how to push people in the right direction and at the right time, because a lot of this stuff is about timing. He's almost like a guardian angel. I can remember being clean and being homeless. You know, I'm clean and I'm homeless and I'm crazy. I didn't want to take anything and I wasn't going to take anything and I was six years clean, and the help that Richard gave me back then invaluable to me. I was in a vulnerable place in my life, and Richard didn't take advantage of me. He just helped me. Richard helped me with shelter, he helped me get a vehicle, and then he helped me get a job, which I'm still at today and have had for over nine years. I went from line staff to associate director at the place I work at. I mean, I wouldn't be who I am today if Richard hadn't come into my life, if God didn't work through him so that I could become somebody I could be proud of. A lot of recovery is being proud of yourself, loving yourself, and spending a lot of time giving others love. Richard has taught me how to be a woman of worth. I remember one day, Richard said to me, "Kim, you are a ten. Why are you conducting yourself like a two?" Straight up! That conversation straightened me out big time. The people you meet and the places that touch your heart change you.

Richard: You know, Kim, I have seen you be a mother to your kids. Even though your kids are grown now, your children are still your children. And I've seen you show unconditional love not only to your kids, but to other people as well. It doesn't matter if they are clean or not, if they are struggling, I have seen you really support your kids. You are the ultimate mother. You put your cape on, and nobody can stop you when it comes to helping your children.

Kim: That's right. I have three grown sons today, and a lot of my parenting is a living amends. I was always there for them except the time that I went to prison, but a lot of the influence I gave them was not positive. The influence that I am giving them now is nothing but positive, and they are going to be my legacy. That's what I live for. I live for them to step into their greatness. They all live on their own, they all have their own cars, they don't live off their mom, but if they need me, they know I'm there. That is valuable. I give them that hope.

Richard: Kim, if there was one thing you would like to say to all the readers out there, if there was one ending message to the people coming out of the game and coming into recovery, what would you want to tell them?

Kim: Number one, know who you are. Two, never give up on yourself, and you can be whatever you want to be. This world has everything to make or break you. You make sure you choose the path.

CHAPTER 7

Sandpaypa

I have someone I just had to put in this book. He brings so much to San Francisco's recovery community: Laron Sanders, a.k.a. Sandpaypa. This man right here is one of my Men in Motion brothers. He came in real young, and he's been clean for twenty-four years now. Laron was twenty-five years old when he came into recovery, and he's been going strong ever since.

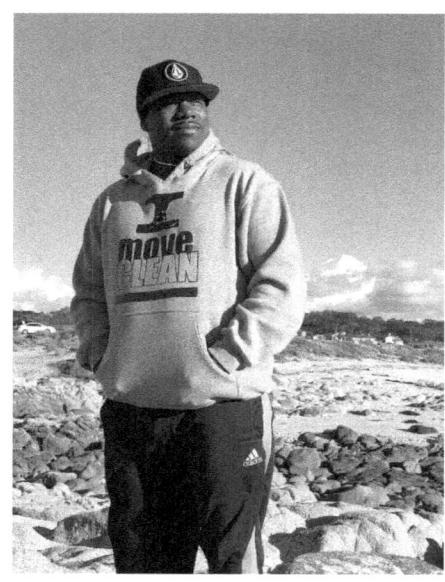

Sandpaypa

Laron: I was nineteen years old when I tried getting sober the first time, but I was twenty-five when I decided to stay.

Richard: When I met Laron in Men in Motion, I was just amazed by how young he was when he came in. He is a musical artist, and he put me in his videos. He actually came out with a video for his tenth anniversary called, "Damn it feels good to be clean." For twenty-four years I have had the pleasure to watch him grow in recovery, and any time I do a recovery event I always call Laron to perform. Thank you, Laron, for your time, and let's get this started.

Laron: Well, I came up in the Fillmore, but I was always against standing on the street and doin' my hustle. I was more of the type that liked to move around a lot. I liked driving my car around and making my money that way. Coming up though, I kind of migrated all over the city but the Fillmore is my home. I hustled. That's how I really made my mark. Everybody used to call me The Sandman; some people in the neighborhood still do call me The Sandman. As an artist I couldn't go by The Sandman because another artist from the other side of town came out as Sandman before I did, so I started using the name Sand-paypa as my artist's name.

I hit my bottom going to jail. When I was young, if I stayed out of jail for sixty days that was good for me. But one of the last times I was in jail, I had done two years and change and I got out for like, eight days, and in those eight days my cousin tried to put me on. I was running between Fillmore and the Tenderloin, and I came out of a hotel room with rocks in my mouth. The police were raiding the hotel, and the nark was trying to talk to me while I was coming out of the hotel. I tried to talk to the nark with the rocks in my mouth, but when I turned around the nark and a couple police started choking me until I spit out the rocks. Once I spit out the evidence, I caught the case, I caught the violation. They dropped the case and gave me the violation, and with the violation they had me go into a treatment center. When I went into the treatment center, they told me I was going to dry out and then they were going to send me to a six-month treatment program. At the treatment center, I was sent to this men's group, and that's where I met Richard Beal. Every Wednesday I would go to this men's group, called Men in Motion. One of my homeboys from my neighborhood was already in the Men in Motion group, and he would become my first sponsor. I trusted this guy because he was from the street like me. I got locked into Men in Motion, and I connected with Richard and my sponsor, and we have all been rockin' together ever since. Today a lot of us work for some of the same companies, some of us are DJ's and we play at each other's recovery events, some of these guys play my songs at their events, we all support one another.

Richard: Laron, can you go back a little bit and talk about how we originally met? Did we meet at Men in Motion, or did we first meet at Milestones, the NA meeting on Fridays? That Milestones meeting was a big part of our relationship too, we had a lot of people going to that meeting. You, me, and Lavell, Rodney, Rod, and a gang of people used to go to that Milestones meeting on 5th Street.

Laron: Yeah, I definitely went to that meeting. There was a Sunday meeting that was really big as well. When I first got into the treatment center, this was this dorm area and everybody used to say, "Man, this is a life-or-death program." But at the time, when I first got into treatment, I wasn't really trippin' like that yet. I didn't see what the big deal was, because I thought I was different when I first came in, right. I still had some hustle in me, and some of these cats were old to me. I still felt like I had the game goin' on inside me, so I didn't get what their deal was in the beginning. But there was this one cat, he was going back and forth with somebody else. This guy caught a feeling and went out, he left the program and he went up to Market Street. He OD'd and he died. About thirty minutes after that argument he'd been having, the police came back to the treatment center and said, "Hey man, this guy OD'd, and he's dead." And that's when it hit me that this *is* a life-or-death program. We are each one bad decision away from dying, and that's when I woke up and knew I needed to change everything inside and out. Also, it only takes fifteen seconds to catch fifteen to life. We've had members who went out and decided to do some bad things, and spent those fifteen seconds, and caught fifteen to life. I finally learned that it's not just about using, it's about my life choices. It's about the decisions I make in my life and the track my life is on.

I continued going through the program, but I ended up getting kicked out of the program for threatening someone when I had about nine months. I was trying to get to my service commitment on time, and one of the desk clerks at the treatment center wouldn't let me get through the line of people so that I could get to my service commitment. Everybody in line offered to let me cut in line so I could get to my commitment, but the desk clerk told me that I couldn't cut and I had to get to the back of the line. So I said something like, "Man, that type of stuff would have gotten your jaw broke on the streets." The desk clerk told the building management that I threatened to break his jaw, but I didn't say I would break his jaw. I said something similar, but I never threatened him directly. They kicked me out of the treatment center for my comment, but Men in Motion came through for me. After my second night at a shelter, a Men in Motion member called me and told me I could stay at his house. All the brothers from Men in Motion were very supportive during that time. More Men in Motion guys called me and told me where to go. I went to the Salvation Army, who put me in transitional housing. I stayed at a halfway house for a minute.

I still wanted to hustle back then, I still wanted to be in the game, but I knew my product had to change. I could not sell what I was selling anymore. My old ways would put me back into the penitentiary, or would get me hooked on the dope again. Like they say, "A monkey can't sell bananas, right." I had to do something different. I was watching Richard and other guys get into new legal businesses, and a lot of the brothers in Men in Motion had their own thriving businesses. They had good jobs, they had families, they got married, and whatever struggles they had, they would bring it to the circle. I was shaped and molded by this circle of great men. We had a brother from the circle who sold FUBU Clothing out of his car. When I saw that, I said, "Man! I could sell clothes too! I could do that." Another brother from the circle had some studio equipment, and he got me into his studio with some platinum artists, I was put in the right place at the right time, and I ended up getting my songs recorded. We cut a record, and I was able to get out there and sell my record, perform on different stages around the country with other well-known artists in the industry, and my lost dreams were awakened. New possibilities arose, and I was able to take my music to the street and make money off it just like I used to do with drugs. I made clothes, I turned myself into a brand that I could be proud of. Eventually, everyone in my family and everyone from my neighborhood started to say, "Man, SanPayPa flipped the game!" I was able to flip the game. I took the game that I learned in the streets and applied it in a positive way, in a legal way. I could finally take my own brand, market it, and distribute it to make money. This was my dream, and I did it. I always wanted to make something that uplifts people, something that motivates and inspires people. Over the years, man, people have come up to me and said, "Man, damn it feels good to be clean, that song got me through some hard times!" People would come up to me in a parking lot in the Fillmore and say, "Man, this song on your album, it helped me get through some dark times. My father just passed, and you helped me." I didn't sell a million records or make a million dollars off of my art, yet, but I have helped uplift people's spirits. I have helped change people's minds. I have changed people's trajectories in life. Art and music can be very powerful, and people have told me that I make powerful music. By telling my story with music, I have been able to make a difference in my community.

All the things that I have been doing with music have put me in line with the things that Richard has been doing with the community. He's been rubbing shoulders with the mayor and the recovery community, and he's been getting people into treatment. I am a little piece of this big umbrella that Richard has opened really wide for so many people. Everything that Richard does has been a motivation and an inspiration for me, like maybe one day I can have a transitional house,

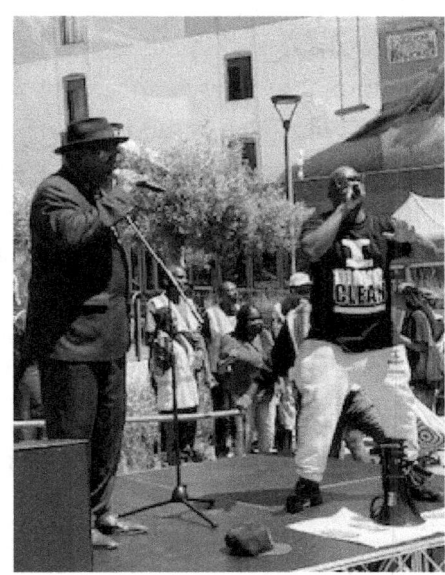

Sandpaypa performing at Recovery Day

maybe one day I can have a treatment program that brothers can come into so we can treat their addiction or their alcoholism, maybe we can give them an alternative to the game they are living in. Richard and I found an alternative, so maybe I can help more people find an alternative.

Richard: Laron, will you tell us how you came up with your song, "Damn, it feels good to be clean?" Tell us how you come up with all of your great songs. And what's the name of your business that you have now?

Laron: Well, when I came up with "Damn, it feels good to be clean," I was coming up on my ten-year sober anniversary. A lot of my music at the time was street, and I had done one song with a couple of other artists called "Fillmore Formula." That was a neighborhood song, right. I wanted to represent The Fillmore. We did a video for "Fillmore Formula." When we finished "Fillmore Formula," I wanted to turn a new leaf and make something different. I wanted to make a song that would represent my upcoming anniversary. At that time, a lot of men in Men in Motion, like Richard and my late, great sponsor Jessie, used to say, "Man, it feels good to be clean!" I would pray to my higher power for an inspirational message to put in music, and I came up with, "Damn it feels good to be clean." I ended up making that song, but CDs had really gone out of style. It was the end of the CD era, so I needed to find a way to sell my new song. I did make some CDs, but then I made a shirt that said, "Damn, it feels good to be clean." I threw a ten-year celebration, and I sold some CDs, and sold my t-shirts, and the t-shirts sold out immediately. The shirt made my song pop.

That night was amazing. We threw a big celebration in the Fillmore on Golden Gate Avenue at an apartment complex. I broke out and performed, "Damn, it feels good to be clean." After that event, I went down to East Palo Alto to a large sober event, and DJ Craig played my song. From that moment on, I couldn't keep up with CD and t-shirt orders. My song blew up all over the Bay Area after that. After that song I made "My gratitude speaks." That song is just raw. It talks about what it takes to be grateful for where I came from and grateful for another day clean, and trying to inspire those who are struggling to stay clean. Then I came up with, "I move clean," because people on the street were always saying, "I move mean" and "I'm out here moving mean." I couldn't say that I was moving mean because I'd left my old game behind, but I could say, *I move clean*. So that's how "I move clean" came out. I posted that song on social media, and before I made any shirts everybody on my social media was asking when I was going to make shirts for "I move clean"? So, I made the "I move clean" shirt, and that shirt did even better than the "Damn, it feels good to be clean" shirt. *I move clean* has also become the name of my brand, so everything I do today goes under the umbrella of "I move clean." Today my message and my brand reach more than my recovery crowd. People who do not live a sober lifestyle also like my brand, and they buy my music and my clothing today. I want my message to reach everybody, and I have succeeded at achieving that goal.

After "Damn, it feels good to be clean" and "I move clean" hit, I came out with "Out here clean." "Out here clean" is another song and design combo that I came up with, and it's about people saying, "Man, I'm out here! I'm outside and I'm out here clean and living my best life." Then I came out with a song called "Hella clean." But at a sober event in San Jose I saw that someone else had already come out with a "Hella Clean" shirt, so I didn't come out with a "Hella Clean" shirt to go with my song. Even without a shirt, that song did really well too.

All this music, and all the recovery, and meeting all the people that I have been able to meet along the way from this big community, have saved my life and changed how I look at the world and everything that goes on around me. All of these things I am talking about have given me something to live for, and they have given my life a purpose. So I continue to crank out more positive songs, and I am trying to bring all this work into a more widespread community. My music isn't for just the recovery community, but for anybody who is struggling for any reason. My message is for anyone who wants to find another way to live, a better, healthier way to live, right. I am trying to put the messages into my songs that I have learned from my brothers in Men in Motion and all those recovery meetings that I have been to over the past twenty-four years. If someone is dealing with depression or anxiety, I want my music to help them. A lot of people lately have been asking me why I don't become a Christian rapper, but I don't want to reach a limited amount of people. My music is for Christians, but my music is also for anyone else who is not a Christian, too. It doesn't matter where you come from. Everybody deserves love. Everybody deserves a good life. My message is limitless, man. I want to surround myself with people who want to change the world. I can't afford to judge and discriminate. I can't say, "Oh, man, you're not in recovery. I can't mess with you." When I see someone crying out for help, that is an open door for me. Guys like Richard have helped me to see when someone is crying out for help.

Richard: You said you came in the first time at nineteen and you were finally able to get clean and stay clean when you were twenty-five. What happened between nineteen and twenty-five?

Laron: When I was nineteen, I went to treatment. The judge gave me a deal where I could go to treatment for eighteen months or do three years in the penitentiary. I chose treatment so I could take what I thought was the easy way out. I looked at treatment as a "get out of jail free card," right. And then when I went into the program, I didn't really do anything that you would do if you were serious about staying clean. I didn't get a sponsor, I didn't work the steps, I just thought that the treatment center would treat me for my addiction, and once I was treated for my addiction, I would be well. I had no idea what any of this stuff was or what it meant. I didn't know recovery was a way of life. When I got out of treatment, I got back into the game because the game called me. I didn't want to change yet. I thought I could be that monkey selling bananas. But once I peeled one banana, I couldn't peel too many bananas more before I took a bite. That put me back in the game and the streets for another four or five years. During my eighteen months in the treatment program, I had not had a drink. When I got out I thought I could drink like a normal person since I'd just been in treatment for a year and a half. I thought I could smoke a little weed without any problems. But I'm not normal. I can't just drink a couple beers and smoke a little weed and put it down. Once I decided to start indulging in the drink and the weed, my addiction ended up getting the best of me, and it happened quick. I came back when I was twenty-five and was ready to surrender to the program. I decided I was going to do everything that people told me to do. At first, I wanted to show everybody that the program didn't work, but I have been doing it for the last twenty-four years and it ain't failed me yet!

Richard: That's what I'm talking about, man. Laron, that was amazing, man. What would you like to tell someone that is just getting into treatment at a young age just like you did? If you had a message for that young person, what would you want to say to that person?

Laron: That message would be, keep your hustle but change your product. *You* are the product.

CHAPTER 8

Roland Williams a.k.a. "RoDog"

O k, everybody, today I have Roland Williams. Roland is a relapse prevention specialist, an interventionist, and a licensed therapist. He's my sponsor, my friend, my mentor, my life coach, and his credentials go on and on. Roland, thank you so much for being here, and thank you for being my sponsor for the last fifteen years. I became a certified relapse prevention specialist because of Roland. Roland is the man who taught me that it doesn't matter how you get here, how you get clean. It's about what you do when you get here that counts. Roland got started in the recovery game while he was in jail and now, many years later, Roland has opened up programs and traveled all over the world helping people. I call him *International Roland*. But Roland's street name for many years was RoDog.

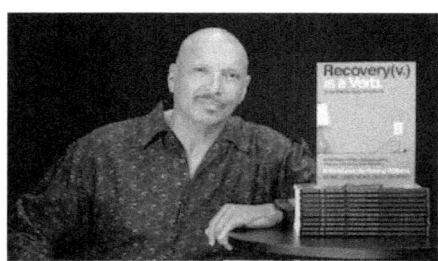

**Roland Williams' workbook,
Recovery Is a Verb**

So, Roland, go ahead and tell us your story, talk about how you got here, your journey, how you found your way to San Francisco, how we connected. It's all you, man. Tell your story.

Roland: Well, first of all I think this is a beautiful, pow-

99

erful, pertinent conversation for so many of us, especially men of color but not just men of color. So many people get caught up in this lifestyle we are talking about. A lot of us get caught up in that part of the lifestyle that we used to call *the game*, and that includes pimpin' and sellin' dope, stick up boys and that whole fast money lifestyle. I think it is important to mention just how addicting this lifestyle is.

I grew up in the South Side of Chicago. In the city. In the hood. You know, I didn't come from the suburbs of Chicago. I didn't come from the mixed neighborhoods. I grew up straight up in the hood on 63rd Street. Anybody who knows that area knows that you could drive all day and never see a white person. You might see a white police officer or a white store owner, but you never saw white people just walking around in my neighborhood. When I was a kid, none of us in my community wanted to be doctors, lawyers, or dentists. We wanted to be players. We wanted to be straight players. We were drawn to the game from the beginning. I remember guys in my neighborhood, like the Great Joe Jones, and Big Shot, guys like Cigar James. And man, I wanted to be like those guys. Big Shot used to pull into the neighborhood in a big ol' Cadillac, with a big ol' ring on his pinky finger, and two big ol' thick girls with the phat booties and the stockings with the line in the back. Big Shot would walk out all of us kids, and he would give us a dollar apiece. Back then you could go see three movies for thirty-five cents. There would be ten, fifteen, twenty kids all standing around Big Shot, and he would just peel off money, and all of us kids would go to the movies together. So yeah, I wanted to be just like Big Shot. All my life I aspired to be part of that crew. I aspired to be hip, slick, and cool, as they say in the rooms. So that's what I chased. I chased that lifestyle.

I wound up going into the military at sixteen, underage, just trying to get out of Chicago. I had a crooked recruiter, and I wound up going to Germany. One weekend I found myself in Amsterdam, and I stuck a needle in my arm for the first time. That was the beginning of my real drug addiction. Sixteen years old, I'm an IV heroin addict. I would tell all those people in the military, "Look, I was just sixteen years old when you all let me in. You need to send me home." They wanted me to come into work every day, but I wanted to shoot dope every day. They sent me home to Chicago at sixteen with an honorable discharge and a $200 a day heroin habit. It was hard to keep that habit going, because the dope in Chicago wasn't as good as that European dope. Plus, Chicago was cold. The day after Christmas in 1976, I decided I needed to be somewhere warm. So me and my partner, my buddy I grew up with, we got on a Greyhound bus seeking warm weather and squares we could take advantage of. We were going to come to California and turn California out. We were going to show those squares how to get paid, how to get money. We were going to show them how to get down, Chicago style. I got off the Greyhound bus on 6th and Market in San Francisco, and it was cold as fuck. I thought we were coming to some palm trees and sunshine. I didn't do any research on San Francisco, and I thought all of California was like Los Angles. I was eighteen or nineteen years old at the time. Well, San Francisco was cold as fuck on the day I arrived. But a guy walked up to me and said, "Hey man, you want a joint?" I said, "Hell yeah!" My partner that I arrived in San Francisco with got into the square life, and he got himself a little square girlfriend. While my buddy got into the square life, I got into San Francisco's underworld. San Francisco's underworld in the '70s, man, it was on and crackin'. George Moscone was the mayor back then, and if you didn't shoot anybody or hurt anybody, you were never going to the penitentiary. The whole scene, The Fillmore, Divisadero, that whole area back then, was just hoes and pimps and dope dealers. We had taken over that whole fucking city. We had a spot at 441 Ellis Street, where it was like New Jack City. We had that whole building at 441 Ellis Street, and it was nothing but hoes and dope dealers and pimps and hustlers. I was so excited to be a part of that life, it wasn't even funny, man. And I was good at this lifestyle. I was good at gettin' money. I was so good at the game, I could talk a cat off a fish wagon. I had a couple of girls, you know, I was three and four deep. I was wearing silk shirts and reptile shoes and I was gettin' high every day. I thought I was livin' the life. I have to tell you, for those first five years I loved every moment of that lifestyle. I slept during daytime and hustled at night. I'd be up for two or three days at a time, and everybody knew me by what I was wearin' and what I was driving. I had a red Cadillac Coup Deville, and on the side door in gold letters, it said *RoDog*. That's what people called me. "RoDog! There goes RoDog!" because I was a dog, right. I was a scandalous, triflin', manipulating, lying hustler. You couldn't trust me worth a damn. That was my claim to fame.

That, and that I was pretty. I was good looking. I was light skinned with curly hair, and that was the bomb back then. So I could catch. There was a guy named Bunny who had a club in the Haight-Ashbury called the Anxious Asp, and that was the spot. I used to go down there and just pluck all those girls one by one. I could catch like a champ back then. But what happened to me was the dope stopped working. Where I once had it going on, I started becoming more dishonest and scandalous. I started slippin' up. I started spending all my money on dope. I stopped paying rent. The dope just gradually squeezed everything out, so by the time I was twenty-five years old I was washed up. I was already a has-been. People started talking about how I used to be this big-time player and how I used to have the nice car and the nice place. Everybody started to see me in the past tense. To keep up with my habit I started selling my jewelry and my reptile shoes, and I started telling my girl to stop by the dope house on her way home and to bring the dope straight home to me. I was embarrassed for people to see what I had become.

I remember one day I went to get some dope, but I was short. My dealer, St. Luise Charles, was from St. Louis. Let me tell you, I had already seen my dealer three or four times that day, and I was short this one time. I said, "Hey man, give me a hit. I'm $5 short, man." He said, "No man, you can't have that," and I said, "Fuck you! You know I'm good for it." I started begging him for just one hit, right. And I'm used to being the player here. I'm used to being a baller. But my dealer said, "Man, quick acting like an old dope fiend!" Man, I can still remember how humiliated I felt when he said that.

I had an apartment over on 3rd and Jamestown, and one day this girl came over who I had been trying to get at for a long, long time. This beautiful sister actually came by my place. But I was dope sick, waiting for my girl to come with some money and some dope. When I got to the door, I peeked through the window and saw this girl that I've been lusting after for months. She had that look in her eye saying, "Hey I'm ready big daddy, I'm good to go." All I could was close the door on her. I was so ashamed. I was so embarrassed. I didn't want nothin' at that time. I didn't want her. All I wanted was some dope.

So, fast forward, I became so scurvied and triflin' at the end, all the hip, slick, and cool was gone. The dope had washed it right off of me. At the same time, my girl and I, we had a son together. My son was my motivation to get clean in the beginning. I tell this story all the time, but one day, I was sitting in my car with no gas in it, just looking out at the San Francisco Bay. I looked in the backseat at my son, and I asked God for help. I realized that if I didn't get clean, he didn't have a chance. And right after that prayer, I went out and caught four felonies that same day. The cops were going to take us all to jail, and they said, "If you don't want this baby to go to CPS, you need to call somebody to come get it." The only number that I knew by heart was the dope man. So, I called the dope man, and his sister came and got my son. That day ended up being the beginning of my journey into recovery.

I ended up doing a year in county, and then they had me go to an eighteen-month program. I came to the San Francisco County Jail in San Bruno, where Richard Beal was working, and Richard gave me an opportunity to speak to incarcerated men inside the facility. I'll forever be grateful for that, because the last time I'd used was right outside that San Bruno facility. June 10, 1986, is my sobriety date, and I've been clean ever since. This past June I celebrated thirty-eight years clean.

But while I was in the program, I was still addicted to the game. I had pictures of all my girls up on my locker, so everybody knew what kind of player I was, how I got down, right. I was fucking everything in the rooms. Before I got clean, I didn't even like sex. I thought anybody that really needed sex was a trick or a square. I could take it or leave it. I preferred dope over sex at any time of the day. But then I came into the rooms, and an NA girl gave me a hug, and my body woke up. I was a tramp in the rooms for a while. I was still hustling: I was stealing from people, and I would steal what other people said and I'd say the same thing. I didn't have any work experience, so I couldn't get a job. Before getting clean, my job was getting money in any way necessary. But in 1986 you didn't need any credentials to be a counselor in California, so I became a counselor. I started working as a counselor when I had six months clean. I was *carrying* the message way before I *had* the message.

To fast forward a bit, I realized at about thirteen months abstinent that I didn't know what the fuck I was doing. I felt like I was an impersonator in recovery. You know, I used to sell bunk dope at the end of my addiction. I would use the real dope and sell the fake dope to the suckers. For a while I felt like I was selling bunk recovery in the rooms. I was faking it. And it occurred to me thinking about these people I'm working with as a counselor, carrying the message I don't even have, that I could actually hurt somebody. For some reason something happened, and I started to develop a conscience. I started developing some remorse. I started to feel like I didn't want to be the bad guy anymore. I didn't like being a taker.

A therapist in the program actually became a role model to me. This brother went back to school in his forties, and he started this program I was in. He was slicker than Richard and I put together, and this guy was using all his game for something positive. And I thought, "Damn, this must be cool. Slick as you are to be doing something positive with it." I wanted to be like this guy, whose name was Richard Lindsey, and he was a therapist at the VA Center. I put myself on a mission to transfer some of my game into something positive. All that same drive and determination that I had when I was young and hustling in the streets, I would take that same energy and skillset to help other people get sober. And after some time, everything started to come together. I started surrounding myself with people that was about this clean life. People were starting to come up to me and pull my coat tail and say, "Hey man, that shit you're doing is played out. You need to check this out. *Here* is the bomb, over here. You know, you need to check out these meetings, you need to check this recovery stuff out. If you're sick of going to jail, then quit doing that shit. We found a way out." I still didn't know that addicts like me got clean. I didn't know that people who were addicted to the life, who were knee deep into it like me and Richard Beal and addicted to the drugs, I just didn't know anybody that was out of that. Nobody came to the TL to 12-step me. There were no programs down there yet. There was no police station in the TL back then. There wasn't anything but us: addicts, pimps, hoes, and hustlers. That's all there was. We had a little community—there was some honor in the game back then. So, anyway, I found myself in recovery, and it resonated with me. I found out that maybe I *could* do this. It took me about nine months clean to realize I wasn't a dog anymore. I was starting to care about people. I found out that it wasn't the messenger, it was the message.

Before recovery, if you weren't a part of the life I came from, the game, you couldn't tell me shit. I wasn't listening to no squares. If you didn't live like me, use like me, I wasn't going to listen to a word you had to say. And that made for a miserable existence. But like I said, it all started to come together in the program. Recovery was working. I started listening to different kinds of people. I started hanging out with different kinds of people, and I found out that there was a lot of us that were tired of the life, tired of the game. The dope kicked our ass. The game kicked our ass. There ain't no retirement plan, no dental plan, no health plan in the game. That life is designed only to kill you. I'm watching all these old players fall by the wayside. Pimps with no hoes. Bikers with no bikes. Drug dealers with no drugs. I started to see behind the scenes, and it wasn't as glamorous as I thought it was.

I got clean right around the time crack came around. When crack came around, people really started to change. There wasn't any more honor in the game. Things got dark. It used to be, you don't take another man's woman, you don't openly disrespect another man on the street, you know, there were rules. But with crack there were no more rules. So, at this time I started gravitating toward a different type of person.

I'd like to talk about you for a minute, Richard. I'll just say that in my career I got on a mission, and I've been able to do some incredible stuff. I've been all over the world, I've written books, I got my story in the Narcotics Anonymous Basic Text. I teach, too, and in the last year I've been going in and out of the California prisons training lifers. I have classes with fifty and sixty prisoners who are all doing life, so I've got guys in my class that have been in prison just as long as I've been clean. You know, one bad decision and it's a wash. These guys in there, they've been locked up for twenty-five to forty-something years. And all it does is remind me of how blessed and lucky I am, and guys like Richard Beal are, all the guys like us who have made it out into this new world of recovery. It could have easily been me and Richard Beal and a lot of other guys we know who could be in prison right now. It's cool to be with people who have that kind of history and who have made it out. That's why I think this book Richard is working on is so important. People need to know there's a way out.

My first couple years that I got clean, I always had nice cars. I used to always drive a Mercedes or a Cadillac, a BMW, a Bentley, and you know what I would do? I would cruise through the TL, clean, leaning, with my jewelry, perpetrating like I used to do back in the day because I missed the way everybody used to look at me. I used to pull up in one of them cars with my jewelry on looking like a player, looking like a hustler but I was clean, working as a counselor. I would creep out there just to remind myself of that feeling. How intoxicating, how seductive that feeling was, to have people look at you the way they look at you when you pull up on the corner. One of them wannabe players walk across the street, and they see me, a real player. But really I'm a counselor. That's how addicted I was to that shit, man, I was still chasing that. My head still told me to do shit that I ain't had no business doing. Like, I'd have a pocket full of money, and my head would tell me to steal something. My head would tell me that I'm an outlaw. I wanted that power, I wanted to get away with some shit. I wanted to do it my way.

I had to unlearn all of these things, and I did. Now I've got a square wife, love her to death, and we've been married for thirty-four years. I got two sons. That boy that was in the backseat of that car I talked about, and another son that we have been able to raise. They ain't never seen their daddy in jail. One of them ain't never seen me high. My wife has never seen me drink or take a drug, and my oldest son doesn't remember me the way I used to be. I found out recently that I have a daughter, too. I have a forty-six-year-old, beautiful daughter. When she found me she needed a dad, and I was able to be there for her. I was able to step up and be the father that this beautiful girl never had in her life. I got four grandkids, I got a whole career, and I feel free of the game. I do sometimes feel the tug. I still dress, I still wear jewelry, I still wear nice watches, and I still drive nice cars. And that's because I like nice stuff. I work hard, so I like to have the nice things that come with hard work. There's still a little hint of who I was in there.

Richard and I have known each other most of the time that Richard has been clean. And Richard is brilliant. Richard has one of the sharpest minds that I know. One of the things that I loved about Richard from the beginning is that he has always been authentic. When I first got clean, I was afraid that I would turn into a square. I was afraid I would become a sucker. I didn't want to be one of them *Leave It to Beaver* motherfuckers. In my mind I always identified as a player. I watched Richard still talking shit, still hustling. He used to hustle out the back of his car. Richard hustles in everything he does. He was a gambler, he was a player, but he was also committed to his recovery. Richard was learning as much as he could, he was helping as many people as he could. Richard wanted to be effective. Richard can reach people that nobody else can reach because of his authenticity. Richard will pull up sharp as a tack, three-piece suits, suited and booted, sharp as a motherfuckin' tack. He'll say, "Look, this is me, this is who I am. I ain't going to put cut on it for y'all. I'm not going to shrink to fit you motherfuckers. I'm Richard

"Dollar Bill." And then Richard has the gift of gab, he's such an amazing storyteller I could listen to him for a long, long time. People might think, if they didn't know Richard, "This motherfucker is really arrogant and he's really into himself." But actually, Richard is quite humble. I have had the privilege of knowing Richard pretty well for a long time now, and yeah, he likes to dress, finesse, and he likes to make people laugh, and he likes to entertain people, but he is actually one of the realest people that I know. Richard will talk about what's going on with him. He asks for help when he needs to ask for help. He takes direction, and he is always doing service for other people. Richard has supported my career ever since I've known him, and he has supported so many other people. He has done so much in San Francisco for all these people, the politicians, the legal professionals. Like when Richard Beal calls on someone, they come. No matter where they are from, they will show up. Richard always thinks outside the box, so he's looking for all different kinds of ways to make a difference. As a result, he's become very accomplished both in the recovery field and in the professional field. There ain't too many people out there doin' it like Richard does it. I don't know anybody else in the Bay Area who has had more of an impact on the black community, on the justice-involved population, and on the drug-addicted community than Richard Beal. Richard has done this by being true to the new game, living sober and being of service.

I've watched Richard go through some ups and downs. I've watched him get challenged. I've watched him get pushed to the limit. But like Richard always says, "Where's your third step now?" Well, Richard has a third step. He's got some tools, and I've watched him use them. And yeah, Richard still has a little "Dollar Bill" in him, and he can still slip back into some old thoughts, but he catches himself. Whenever I think about Richard, I smile. Richard is a good brother, and I'm proud to know him. He's a shaker and a mover. Richard has my support from now on, til the wheels fall off.

Richard: Amazing, man, thank you. Roland, if there was one thing that you would like to say to the community, to the TL, if there was one thing that you would like to say about recovering from the game, what would that be?

Roland: Well, what I'd really like to say is that the game will kill you, man. You know, it almost killed me. My addiction to the game almost ended me. For the longest time, I didn't know that people made it out of the game. Just know that there is another way. There is a whole other life waiting for you.

CHAPTER 9

Men in Motion

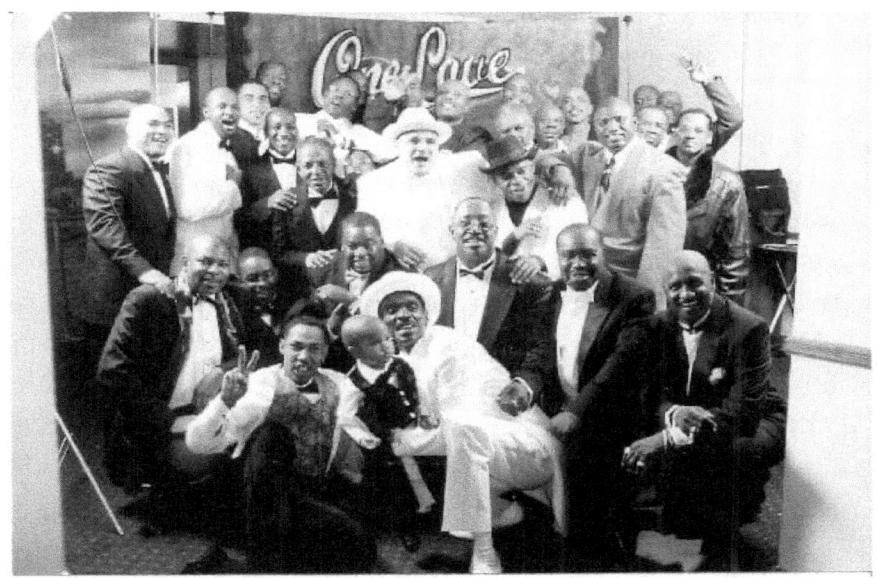

Men in Motion

You know, I have been thinking about creating this book for the past ten years, but I could not write a book about recovery without talking about Men in Motion and the impact it has had on my recovery. Men in Motion was a men's support group that started at Glide Memorial Church here in San Francisco in the late 1980s. Before Men in Motion, there was another support group at Glide called Facts on Crack, right when the crack epidemic exploded in the Bay Area. In the late '80s, crack was everywhere. Murder rates went up because addicts would do anything and everything for crack cocaine. I went to Facts on Crack meetings, and at that time all I knew was that I was an addict. I knew I had the disease of addiction, but I didn't know what that really meant yet. I hadn't read the chapter out of the Big Book called The Doctors Opinion. The Doctors Opinion talks about the lack of control that someone like me has when it comes to drugs and alcohol. An addict like me can't control how much I use once I start. In my mind, crack was the problem. If I could just get off this crack, I'd be good. I used to go to the Facts on Crack meetings and then go across the street to Boeddeker Park and smoke weed. I did this until I went to Men in Motion, which was started by this guy named Jesse Primm, who eventually became my first sponsor. Jesse would say to me, "Man, you gotta check out Narcotics Anonymous, because Narcotics Anonymous talks about complete abstinence from all drugs." Before Jesse told me about NA, I thought I would be ok if I quit crack and alcohol, but I never thought about marijuana being an issue. I mean, smoking weed was my thing. Smoking weed was my first love, right since I was nine years old. At twelve years old I'd been selling fifty cent joints, five-dollar matchboxes, and three-fifty lids. Again, in my mind, I just needed to get off that crack.

Eventually I met some guys who were teaching classes at Glide, men like Dr. David Smith and Dr. Daryl Nob. Experts knew that something had to be done because of all the people dying from crack cocaine. There wasn't a massive spike in overdoses back then, but crime was going up because people did whatever they had to do to get the money to afford their crack habits. I was one of those people back then. I didn't do all the dark sexual stuff that a lot of other people were doing, but I was doing just about everything else.

I was introduced to Jesse Prim back in 1989. He created Men in Motion with a few other guys, like Mitchell Shelton and Paul Thomas. These guys told me straight up that I needed to stop using. Eventually I went to Men in Motion, and then some of those guys told me I needed to get into Narcotics Anonymous. These were the guys who told me that I could learn about the disease of addiction in NA. I didn't know simple things, like "one is too many" and "a thousand isn't enough" or that substituting one drug for another is just a symptom of the disease.

Once I started going to Men in Motion on a regular basis and got into treatment, my treatment program allowed us to go to one outside meeting of our choice a week. We were mandated to go to the Post and Mason meeting, which was the biggest NA meeting back in the day. We called it the "Big Booty" meeting, because all the girls would get dressed up and show everybody what they got. Then on Tuesday nights was the Saint Mary's Cathedral AA meeting, the biggest AA meeting at that time. So I had Men in Motion, the Post and Mason NA meeting, and Saint Mary's Cathedral AA meetings every week. I begged to go to a meeting every day. I was serious about getting clean and staying clean.

Going to Men in Motion really helped me. The format of Men in Motion was different from NA and AA. Everybody sat in a circle, and we gave a one-minute check in. But if you were going through something big in your life, you could request three minutes to share with the group. After everybody checked in, you got feedback from the other men in the group about your share, and the feedback you got was really good. In AA and NA, you don't receive feedback from anyone. If someone tries to comment on what you share in 12-step meetings, that's considered crosstalk, and crosstalk is a no-no in most 12-step groups. At a Men in Motion group, I would talk about my strained relationship with my mother, and I would talk about my experience being abandoned by my mother. After I shared about my mother, other men in the group would share their experiences with their mother or father and how they dealt with their abandonment issues. Before Men in Motion, I didn't know that there was a place for me to share my feelings on life, other than talking with a counselor. Right away, I loved getting feedback from the other men at Men in Motion meetings, and I loved being able to give feedback to the other men who shared. At NA meetings, some of the old-timers would tell the newcomers that nobody wanted to hear from them. They would say things like, "Take the cotton out of your ears and put it in your mouth." Back in the '80s and '90s, you were an old timer if you were five years clean. So most of the people who talked at NA meetings had five or more years clean.

Another thing I loved about Men in Motion is that every other month we hosted fundraisers and dances, and men and women from all over the Bay Area would come to these events. We'd get all dressed up, and we learned how to have fun together clean. Men in Motion was poppin'. So many people came to meetings, we'd all give quick one-minute shares so everyone could share, and still our meetings would last two and a half to three hours. Nobody wanted to leave until everybody had their turn to check in with the group. A passion was in the air back then. Eventually our meetings got so big that we needed to leave Glide, so we rented that larger space over on 6th Street. Those meetings up on 6th Street were powerful, man. Our meeting would start at 6pm and we'd be in there until 9:00 or 10:00pm. I was the secretary for Men in Motion for eight years. I took all the meeting notes and kept us organized.

Jesse was my sponsor for about ten years. When he had come into recovery, he couldn't read or write. I created all of Jesse's contracts for Men in Motion. For a while, Jesse and I would meet up to do step work together, and after we were done doing step work, I'd write up contracts for Jesse. Jesse and I were really close for many years. Jesse paid me for the work I did for him, and we'd go out to eat, to talk about life and recovery. These early days were imperative to me staying clean. Men in Motion, NA meetings, my relationship with all the other men in recovery and with Jesse were crucial parts of my early recovery. But of course, time goes on and life has to change. The core group of Men in Motion guys moved away; some guys got married, a few relapsed. We lost our building on 6th Street, and even though we talked about getting a 501(c)(3), we never got that up and running. Some of us still met in person once a month, and when Zoom became a thing, some of us would meet on Zoom. We kept hosting an annual fundraiser for a program that we wanted to help out. One year we might raise money for Glide, and the next year we might raise money for the Haight-Ashbury

Free Clinic or Walden House. We spoke at treatment centers all over the San Francisco Bay Area. Treatment centers from around the Bay Area would call us and ask us to stop by and speak on a weekly basis. Dr. Joe Marshall of the Omega Boys Club ran a radio show called "Street Soldiers," and we would get on the radio and speak about recovery. Back then Men in Motion was all over the place, and we were making a real difference.

Jesse and I disagreed on some things when it came to Men in Motion and the growth of Men in Motion. Every year we gave out a Men in Motion Man of the Year Award and had a big celebration. The year I thought I was going to receive the Man of the Year Award, things went a little sideways. The award was between me and a man named Lavell, and when the board voted on who would win the award there was a tie. Jesse was the tie-breaking vote, and of course I thought I was going to win because Jesse was my sponsor. Well, Jesse voted for Lavell, who got the Man of the Year Award, and I fired Jesse as my sponsor on the spot. Lavell was a good brother, but I was doing all this work for Men in Motion. Besides being the secretary, I was doing all this other side work for the group, so their choice to give the award to Lavell didn't seem right to me. Everybody's got a breaking point, and that was mine. The relationship that I had with Jesse was ruined, so I got another sponsor named Darrell, out of Oakland.

When the pandemic hit, I said, "Ok, we used to do Recovery Day in the park, right." Back then it had been just Men in Motion going into Boeddeker Park and speaking, we kept things very simple. We set up a microphone and some speakers, and we just started talking recovery. This was back when people were openly using drugs in Boeddeker Park every day. I used to use dope in Boeddeker Park everyday as well. Shootin' dope, smoking crack, we were all doin' our thing back in the day. So, Men in Motion would set up amongst all the dope fiends and we'd talk recovery. In my mind, Boeddeker Park was still the best spot to send out our message. Just get in the middle of it all.

In 2021, Mayor London Breed declared a State of Emergency in the Tenderloin because of all the drug use and overdoses around the neighborhood. I wanted to bring back Recovery Day in Boeddeker Park, but I wanted to make the new Recovery Day different. We are going to invite more people, give out awards, bring a lot of good food, have bands come out and play great music, and just make it a big ol' thang, right. That was my idea, and that's what I was going to do. This Recovery Day I invented was inspired by the earlier Recovery Days held by Men in Motion. I made sure to call all my brothers at Men in Motion, and I gave Men in Motion the first reward at my first Recovery Day. A lot of my Men in Motion brothers showed up, spoke, took pictures together, and it was a beautiful thing.

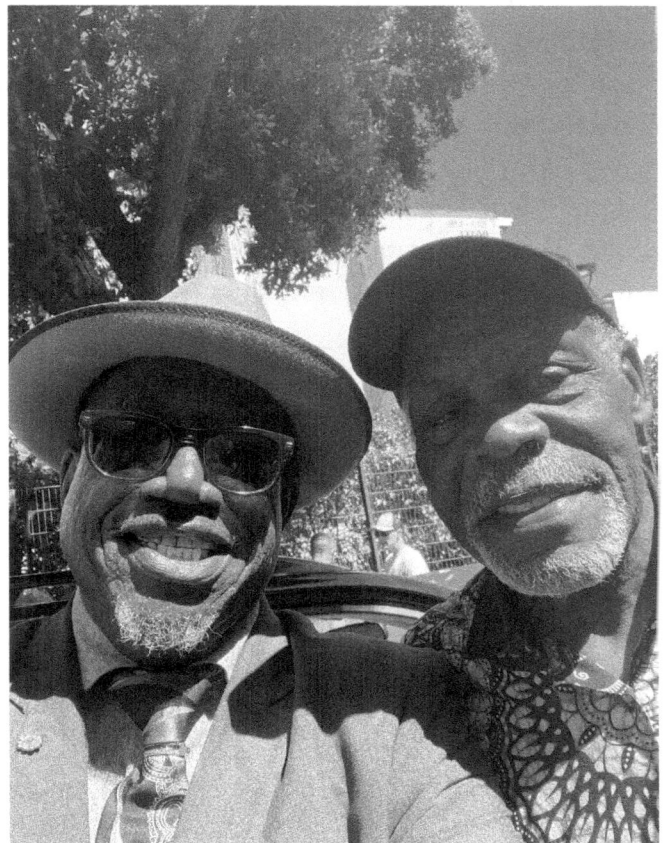

Richard and Danny Glover at the 2024 Recovery Day

I tried to recreate Men in Motion again next door from the Drake Hotel, but that meeting didn't survive for very long. We just couldn't get the traction that the group had back in the '80s and '90s. When we tried starting it back up in 2021, maybe ten people would show up, then it went down to five people, and then three people, and then two people until it just died. Some groups just die, right. A lot of us still keep in touch, still call each other and catch up. We will probably set up a big dance event in 2025, but I don't know if regular meetings will ever come back. Many original members are still clean, with thirty-plus years in recovery, and most of us are committed to going to recovery meetings and helping other people. We're living in different parts of the country, still carrying the message of recovery.

I love what I do today, working in the field of addiction and recovery. I love staying connected with people I met over the years, I love meeting all the new men and women who will become the future of recovery and keep pushing that positive message out to the people who need it and want it. I'll always have so much gratitude for Men in Motion. Men in Motion and the men in that group saved me, and made me the man I am today.

With all that said man, here it is, twenty-nine years later, still clean, still grateful, and still working that same script: Trust God, clean house, and help others.

CHAPTER 10

Dr. Michael Pasley a.k.a. "Fleetwood Mike"

I would like to introduce to you a gentleman named Dr. Michael Pasley. He has a doctorate in theology, and he's pastor of a church. But he is also known as Fleetwood Mike. He's got about thirty-five years clean now. He is the director of the Senior Ex-Offenders Program, a reentry program that works with people coming out of the criminal justice system. Michael has been out here in California for a long time, but he made bones out in New York. Michael and I have been working together for six years now, and he works with the same population of people I work with. His organization received the Recovery Day Award at the 2024 Recovery Day I organized over at Boeddeker Park in the TL. Back in the day, Michael was in the lifestyle out in New York that we have been talking about throughout this book. Then he came out here to California, got clean, and started working with other people who needed help as well. He came from the streets of New York, he went through his journey, and now he is, of course, Dr. Michael Pasley.

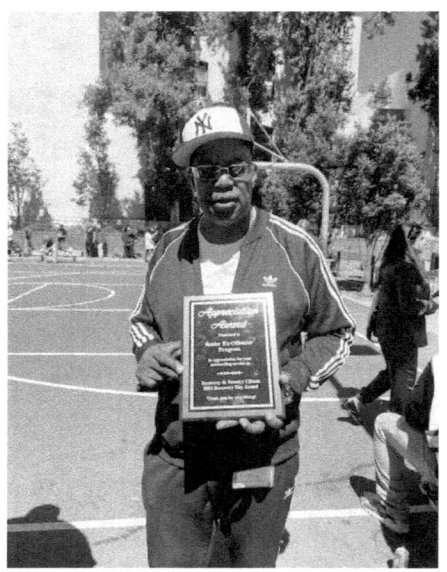

Dr. Mike Pasley, a.k.a. "Fleetwood Mike"

Michael: Well, first of all, let me start off by sayin', with no bragging rights on my past life, I was young and dumb but I had it goin' on. This might seem like an arrogant statement, but I was one of those kids that was fortunate enough to get the forty acres and a mule. I didn't come from a life of livin' in the projects. My family didn't go to jail. And I'm talking about both sides of my family. My father came from a well-established family, my mother as well. My going to the streets was not because of what a lot of other black families have experienced as far as trying to make it in society. I chose to go to the streets.

I actually went into the military at seventeen years old, after I finished high school. Matter of fact, the thing that took me to the military was that my father wanted me to go straight to college. I didn't want to go to college, I just wanted to drive trucks for my father's trucking business, right. My father and all his brothers owned trucks. My very first trip driving a truck, I wrecked that truck. And I'm talking about an eighteen-wheeler. I wrecked my father's eighteen-wheeler. So to avoid college, I joined the military and was sent to Germany. Hash was a big thing over there, and I started selling hash and heroin. I started snorting heroin right away, too. When I came back home to New York, my father was upset because I didn't want to drive trucks anymore. I entered into college, but since my father and I weren't getting along too well, I decided to pack my bags, leave New York, and go to New Haven, Connecticut. That's where my life of pimping and selling drugs really got started. I did this for about five or six years, and finally one day I woke up and I said, "You know what, man, I can't do this anymore."

Richard: Mike, tell us a little bit about how you got turned out with the pimpin' and the game in Connecticut. Who was the guy that turned you onto the game?

Michael: Absolutely. I was around people like Connecticut Slim, Howard Powell, a guy named Derek Carr, you know, guys like that. When I first got to Connecticut, I had a pimped-out Monte Carlo. I parked that car and got myself a Fleetwood, and that's where the name Fleetwood Mike came from. I had the baddest Fleetwood in the state of Connecticut, man. It was a rose pink with white interior and what happened with that? Well, the females just started choosin'. They were choosin' me. And like I said, I was young and dumb. You know, I'm from New York, and those girls just started diggin' on me. The females pretty much turned me out, you know, by choosin' me. I couldn't say no to them, and they couldn't say no to me, right. So, I did all that for a while until I couldn't figure out why I was doing what I was doing with my life. Things started to get pretty wild for me after a while. I had gotten robbed for everything that I had.

Richard: Hey, Michael, tell us a little more about when you got robbed. What was that all about?

Michael: Well, the one thing I can always say, even though I was hustling, I always kept a job on the side. You know, when I started pimpin' I would keep a job *and* pimp. I did quit one of my jobs once and started pimpin' full time, but I got robbed because I went out to get some dope, this fiend pulled me into his house, he robbed me, took my car. I had just freed up all the money I had, so I had a big sack of cash on me, and he got all that too. This was back in 1980, so it was just before crack had come out. After getting robbed, I pretty much gave up full-time pimpin' and hustlin'. I mean, one minute I was ridin' high and then the next minute my car, my money, and all my dope was gone. I did bounce back from that, but I just woke up and realized everything I was doing was wrong. I wasn't getting anywhere with my life, not the way I was living. I was alone in Connecticut without my family, but I had a family business to go to in New York. So I decided to go back to New York in 1981. I stayed there for a bit, straightened my life up, but I got caught up on crack for about six months. I don't mean to say this in a disrespectful way, but I had too much hustle in me to let crack take me out. I guess you could have called me a functioning crack smoker. I was driving my father's truck up and down the East Coast, hauling produce. I would only smoke on the weekends, right. I was a weekend warrior. I'd go buy a sack, I'd have a couple guys go out and sell most of it, and I'd sit at home and smoke the rest. Crack never really had a chance to take me down because I was lucky enough to never smoke the whole bag. And I don't feel good about this, but I was married at the time I was doing all this. I still am married to the same woman. We just celebrated forty years last week.

I stopped smoking crack, but after I stopped smoking crack, I went back to selling and snortin' coke. My wife left me for a while when I went back to coke. When she left me, that was a killer for me. That's what it took for me to want to make a real change in my life. And one thing I don't want to leave out is, when I was smoking crack, I got my wife hooked on crack. But we were too smart and lucky to stay hooked on that dope for long. My wife backed up off the dope we were smoking right around the same time I did. When my wife left me, I moved out to California from New York in 1988. I wanted to show my wife that I could get my life together.

When I arrived in California, I was wearing a size twenty-eight waist pair of Jordache jeans— they were highwaters because they were my brother's jeans and he was shorter than me—and I had one suitcase. I was tore up, man. But I wanted to get my life together, and I knew that I wanted my wife back. Whatever it took to do that, that's what I was going to do. I came out to California because I had a class A license, and I wanted to get into the teamsters. I got to California in January of 1988, and by March I was working driving trucks in San Francisco, making local deliveries for about a year. After that I got a better job driving trucks, and today I get a check on the fifteenth of every month because I'm a retired teamster. I retired from the teamsters in 2002, which is also when I got my first church. I had a really bad experience with the first church I pastored at, so I left that church in 2006. In 2007 another church called me up, and I started pastoring at that church. Financially, we did really well at that church right away, but as gentrification came and kind of killed the city of Oakland, I had to go back to work. This is when I started helping people recover from addiction. I had never done this kind of work before. But I knew that, out of all the dirt that I did, I never went to jail. All the coke I smoked, all the coke I sold, all the people I hurt, I knew that helping other people get clean was a way for me to give back. I had no training in helping people, but I learned from people like Richard Beal. I look at Richard as a mentor. I look toward Debbie Turner as a mentor as well. Debbie is the one who really got me going in the direction of helping people recover. I have been doing this work for about seven years now. I was a case manager at first, and because of my degree in strategic leadership I was able to become the director of our program when a position opened up. I have had a very humbling experience. My life is really simple these days. And there ain't much to me, man. What you see is what you get. I love hard and I fight hard.

Richard: Mike, our stories are similar, how you started off as a case manager for the Senior Ex-Offender Program, and then became a supervisor, and then the director of the program. And your lifestyle is similar to what I came from. I think that's why we have the connection that we have today. You talked about going to Connecticut, the pimpin' and the game, and sellin' dope to keep your habit goin'. That's pretty much my story. You were just doing it on the East Coast and I was doing it on the West Coast. The only difference was your family had a business, and my family business was the game. So I feel connected to you. And Mike, you got heavy into crack for less than a year but as we both know, it don't take long for that stuff to take hold of you and turn you upside down, right.

Michael: Yeah, it don't take long at all. That's right. But yeah, I stopped smoking it but I kept sellin' it, and I kept on with the coke for a while.

Richard: How long have you been clean now?

Michael: I have been off everything since 1991.

Richard: That's what I'm talking about, man. And some people get it through church, some people get it through mentorship, support groups. But it's not how you get it, it's really how you keep it. A lot of people know how to get clean, but a lot of people don't know how to stay clean. It's about staying clean, man.

Michael: Right, absolutely.

Richard: And you got that kind of drive that I got. I can't walk down the street without people stopping me, asking me questions. "Hey Richard, man, it's good to see you man, I need this, I need that, can I get a job, where can I get some housing?' I can't walk a block without somebody stopping me on the street asking me for some type of support.

Michael: Right, well you never know. Somebody might be in a life and death situation.

Richard: That's right man, you just never know. No matter where you go to get your recovery, the spiritual principles are all connected. They are all the same.

Michael: One day, my wife noticed how burned out I was getting. And she said, "Well honey, maybe you should quit that job helping all those people all the time." And you know what I told her? I said, "I'll give up the church before I quit that job." Because it's not the job that burns me out. Believe it or not, I'm tired of the fake people, the people that are in it for the wrong reasons. You know, a lot of people don't know what their calling is. But I know for sure, this work we are doing is my calling. There's people like me and you, Richard, who can reach the people that need our help. We know that the percentage of people who stay clean out there is low, but if we can just reach one or two or three people, it's all worth it. My outlook on life is, God put me on this earth for a purpose, and it's to serve people. And that's what I'm going to do until my last breath. I am a servant. That's my biggest success story.

Richard: You know what, man. You can't end it better than that, man. You know, if you don't know what your purpose is, you allow someone else to dictate your purpose for you. You are truly free only when you find out your true purpose.

Michael: I remember you told me this, the very first time you asked me to speak at Recovery Day. I said, "Man, I don't have the same story that a lot of these fellas have. I wasn't all cracked out on the street for years." But you said, "Yeah Mike, but you were addicted to the lifestyle." And I never forgot that. Because this lifestyle we are talking about is an addiction all on its own. Addiction is just something I figured I would always have to have inside or around me. But none of that is true. Every morning when I wake up, I say, "Lord, put somebody in my path that I can help today." That one prayer is stronger than any addiction that I have ever had.

Richard: That's what I'm talking about! Man, this is why I wanted to talk to you today. Because everybody has a different story. You came to the church, and now you're pastoring the church. Some people went to 12-step meetings, some people do support groups, there are so many options for getting help, getting clean and staying clean. The only thing that matters is recovering from that addiction and setting your life free. The drugs are just *a symptom* of the disease of addiction. I can't say that enough and I can't hear it enough. The disease of addiction can manifest itself in many ways. There are many paths with one destination, and the destination is recovery.

Michael: Absolutely!

Richard: So, thank you man, for being a part of this.

Michael: No, thank you, Richard. And I can't say it enough, man, I love you like a brother, man. You know that.

Richard: I love you too, Michael.

Michael: You know, we hit it off the very first day that we met, and it's been like that ever since. You've just been a solid brother, Richard. I can't say that about a lot of people. My wife will let everybody know that I'm a loner. I don't let a lot of people get close to me, and that's because of the game. I've always had my guard up. But I never felt like that around you.

Richard: Well, man, just so you know, the next lunch is on me, man. You know, we break bread and we fellowship and we talk recovery and we help people. That's what we do. So, thank you again Michael, and I'll be seeing you soon. God bless!

CHAPTER 11

Eric Adams a.k.a. "E Money"

I have a man right here that does more service in Oakland, California, than anybody I know. When the pandemic hit, Eric and I started NA Zoom meetings immediately. I think Eric and I started the first NA Zoom meetings in the Bay Area. There were many times where it was just Eric and me on those meetings, back in the early days of covid. We have also had a business relationship over the years as well. Eric started his own business, and we got connected through the wholesale clothing business. Eric and I have always been about transferable skills, you know, everything is supply and demand. Eric is also a stand-up comedian. I have hired Eric to perform at the Peacock Lounge, even at my wife's birthday party. We go back to when he started recovery, which is about fifteen years or so. I always call him, "E Money," so this is my guy, "E Money." He is one of my closest friends and a great partner of mine. Eric, I want to thank you again for being a part of the project. Tell us how you got into recovery, talk about what it was like for you and what life is like now.

Eric: I grew up in West Oakland, heroin was my drug of choice. I didn't really shoot any dope, I didn't really smoke any dope, but I snorted everything that I ever did. I started using at the age of thirteen, and I didn't stop til I was thirty-eight. When I first attempted to stop using, I went to a program called The West Oakland Health Council, and that's where I learned about Narcotics Anonymous. I wasn't really ready to stop using, I just went there as part of

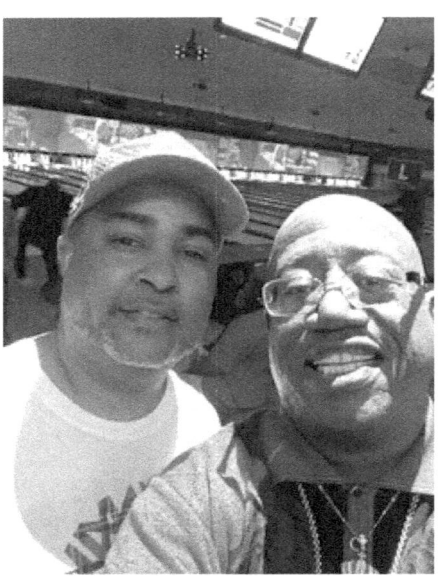

Eric "E Money" Adams and the Ambassador

the methadone program. When I graduated from that program, I went right back to the streets to do what I had been doing. Five years later I went to jail: January 18, 2009. January 19 is my clean date. That's the first day that I went a whole day without any drugs.

When I went to jail, I went to the hospital because in my kick process, it can get really bad. I don't like to kick dope inside general population, right. So I went to the hospital, stayed there for seven days, and when I got out of the hospital, I was put back in general population. Before they were able to search me out and put me in my bunk, I passed out. I woke up with twelve staples in my head. So, I ended up at the hospital again, and the doctor asked me what happened, but I didn't have a memory of what happened or how I ended up on the floor. The doctor told me that I must have been dehydrated from all the diarrhea and throwing up I was doing while kicking heroin in the hospital that past seven days. When I recovered from all that, I got on my knees and prayed. I wasn't praying to get out of jail, I was praying that when I did get out of jail, that God would help me stay clean. I ended up going to court and they offered me eight months, but I didn't take the eight months. I asked them to give me a year, because if you do eight months you have to do it in county. I didn't want to do county time. I'd rather do my time in the penitentiary. I had been in jail for exactly sixty-three days when I went to Superior Court. Before I was let out of the bullpen, I did my little prayer asking God to allow everything to go well, please let them give me this year so I can go do my time and get out of here, and please give me some help when I get out. When I came out of the bullpen, the judge said something to me that had never happened to me before, or to anyone else that I know. The judge pulled out a file and started writing in it. He asked the bailiff to bring me up to the front of the courtroom so he could speak to me directly. At first, I thought I caught another charge. I thought they were going to deny my one-year prison request. But the judge said, "Whatever you were doing back there in that bullpen, you better keep doing that when you get out. Because I have a good feeling that I'm never going to see you again. I'm going to let you go home today." The judge told me that he wrote down that I was on felony probation, and he was going to let me continue on that probation. Then he told me he was going to give me another separate five-year felony probation for the case that had brought me there that day. So I had two five-year felony probations. The judge told me if I ever came back to jail for any reason, I would go back to his courtroom, and if I ever saw him again, I would be going to jail for a very long time. The judge asked me if I could handle the terms I was just given and I told him, yes, I could. He told me to go do what I had to do, and I went home that day. From that point on, I knew God heard my prayers, and I knew God believed in me. This gave me the desire to believe in myself.

I got out of jail and started going to church. I wasn't in NA yet. One day in church I ran into my counselor from the West Oakland Health Council, and she told me that she was on a date with a gentleman who was a regular at my church. And I knew this was a God shot, because my counselor wasn't what you would call a religious person, and she never went to church. My counselor pointed out the man that she was on a date with. She told me that he had been asking to take her out for over a year, and she'd told him if he picked somewhere safe, she'd go out with him. So it was *definitely* a God shot that I ran into my counselor at that church on that day. My counselor suggested that I do some classes with her, to study relapse prevention, recovery dynamics, and anger management. My counselor asked me when I went to an NA meeting last, and I told her it had been about five years since I went to any kind of meeting. She gave me an NA schedule and told me that I should check out some meetings. She told me to go to any meetings on that schedule except for two of them. I asked her, "What meetings should I stay away from?" She said, "400 Broadway and Rumble in the Jungle." And I said, "Why can't I go to those meetings?" And she said, "Pimps, hoes, and gangsters hang out at those meetings!" And I said, "I'm on my way!" As soon as she told me what kind of people frequented those two meetings, I knew I needed to go there. I needed to be around the type of people that I could relate to. People that were like me. My counselor would tell me that not only was I addicted to the drugs, but I was also addicted to the lifestyle. I was addicted to the streets. She told me that I would find a lot of people that come from where I came from at those meetings. So, I went to The Rumble in the Jungle meeting the next night, and the next day after that I went to The 400 Broadway Meeting, and I made that my home group. The 400 Broadway meeting is where I met Richard Beal. Richard's background is similar to mine, since we both come from the streets. I know that Richard is from Richmond and I'm from Oakland, but it's all the same thing in the end. Learning how much clean time Richard had was one of my attractions to him, as somebody who had been in the streets and been in the same type of situations and troubles and hustles. I knew that I could recover if Richard could do it. My process of recovery really started at those meetings.

One of my things back in my street days is I used to boost. That was my main hustle, but I stopped doing all that when I got sober. One day somebody from my home group told me that he and a few guys were going to lunch, and they wanted me to join in. But I said, "Man, I ain't goin' to lunch, I ain't got no money." He said, "Don't worry about it, we got you." All the old timers used to treat the newcomers to lunch, but I was tired of everybody buying me lunch. But he asked, "Why don't you have any money?" and I said, "Because I gave up all illegal activities so I could hang out with y'all at these damn meetings, and I got no job so I ain't got no money." And then he asked me, "So what did you used to do when you were on the street?" And I answered, "I used to boost." He told me that I should keep hustling like I used to hustle, and he gave me the address to the business office where you get your business license. He told me I could buy shit and sell it instead of stealing it and selling it. A lightbulb came on, and the next day I went to down to the office he told me about. I got all the licenses you can have for a clothing business, and I started my first legal business journey that day. I started buying different products, and I found out that a few people in the NA rooms was doing the same thing. Richard was one of them. When I linked up with Richard he really helped me go to the next level with my business. I started learning more about the wholesale process, and I started finding better products to sell. Richard and I have been rockin' like that ever since. Richard has been an inspiration to me not only in the business world, but also in the recovery world. I've always liked how Richard can bend and bounce back from hard times when they come, so they never, ever break him. Richard always comes out on top, and I like to stay close to that.

Richard: Eric, tell us about your transitional house, and how we were able to put together that safe house.

Eric: When I first got into recovery, I had been married for eleven years, with a four-bedroom house in West Oakland. My wife and I were a case of "opposites attract." I was a criminal, boosting, drinking, and doing drugs, and my wife didn't do any of that. She didn't steal, she didn't smoke anything, no drinking, nothing. She just loved me, and to this day I do not know why, but she did. When I got out of jail after those sixty-three days, I went home to my wife, but everything between us was different because we were no long in that "opposites attract" relationship. I had changed. When I got clean, *everything* changed. I ended up calling that same counselor to let her know what was going on, and she recommended a transitional house to me. I went to stay at that transitional house, and ten days after I got there, the guy that was the house manager attempted to relapse. He went to go buy a rock at the local drug house. He went in, bought his drugs, had the clutch fist on his rock. On his way out of the door, the Drug Task Force was coming in. He got caught with his rock in his hand before he was even able to use it. That's why I call it an *attempted* relapse. That guy ended up going to jail. My counselor recommended that I become the new house manager, so the guy who owned the house offered me the job. At first I turned down the offer, but the property owner convinced me to take over the house. I ended up managing that house for two and a half years. When my mother had a stroke I left the job for a year to take care of her, and when she got better, I went back and managed that house for two and half more years. Eventually I moved out and got my own place. Soon after that, I came across another transitional housing building that needed a manager. Working with another guy who was connected to people who needed transitional housing, I made an agreement with the owner, and we started moving people into the building. As of December 15, 2024, my men's home had been open six years. A couple months after that, I celebrated fifteen years that my clothing business has been open, and eight years that I have worked for the city of Oakland for the Department of Violence Prevention. I get to work with troubled teens and victims of violent crimes. I feel like this is a way for me to give back and clean up the streets that I messed up in the past.

Eventually Richard hooked up with me. He started talking about areas of business that I had never heard of before. Richard taught me about nonprofits, becoming eligible for donations, and all the other legal workings of the business world that I didn't know anything about.

Richard taught me how to save my companies money by filing the right paperwork to become a nonprofit. Richard did the paperwork, and I got the nonprofit status. Richard referred me to all the right people who helped me become a full-fledged businessman. I am now in the process of becoming a full charitable organization with the state of California. All I can say is that I am truly living a life beyond my wildest dreams right now. I didn't think someone with my background could have the life I have today, and for that I am truly grateful.

Richard: Eric, can you mention some of the trials you went through during your recovery? I know you have been through some things that would be hard for anyone to make it out of.

Eric: When I was three years clean, my grandmother died. She had been the glue that held the family together. When my grandmother died, it seemed like my whole family just went to their corners, and everybody kind of lost touch with one another. As a kid I used to see my family every day, because everybody would be at grandma's house throughout the week. When she passed away, we all separated from each other. That same year, my son was murdered. Members of the recovery program helped me get through all that loss and stay clean. Staying clean through all that convinced me that I was here, that I was going to stay sober no matter what happened. Prior to all that, in the back of my mind I'd known something was going to come up, I just didn't know what it was going to be. And I hadn't known for sure I could stay clean through such traumatic experiences.

After my son was murdered, I started to experience other deaths within my blood family, as well as some of my friends and other members in the program. My sister passed away from diabetes-related issues. After my sister, my daughter's mother passed away, and after that, my other sister passed away from diabetes-related issues as well. Soon after that, my stepmother—who had been married to my father for fifty years—was gone. My mother's husband passed away shortly after my stepmother. Two years ago, my brother passed away on October 8, on the twelfth anniversary of my son's death. To this day, we don't even know how my brother died. The coroner's office told us that they could only give us two reasons that they know he *didn't* die from. He didn't die from an overdose, and he didn't die from covid, but that's all they knew. Right after my brother, my mother passed away. So, over the years, it has just been one significant death after another. And in between those deaths members of the program lost their kids, lost their parents and others they were close to. Friends of mine who were still in active addiction passed on. A lot of people that I have loved have been comin' and goin' throughout these past fifteen years I have been clean. But I knew when my son passed away and I didn't relapse, I knew I was here, no matter what.

Richard: That's what I'm talkin' about. And you know, Eric's brother Emmit who passed away, Emmit was my sponsee, too. Eric and I have been close for a long time now. We are close with each other's families: I know Eric's kids, and Eric was there when my wife Gerri passed away. Eric and I have seen and been through a lot together. When you are in the middle of major things happening in your life, you just don't know what's going to happen. Eric was one of those guys, when he first came into the rooms of recovery, you just didn't know if he was going to stay clean or not. But Eric is one of those guys who stays clean.

I think what also kept Eric and me sober is that we found ways to be creative in our recovery. In the beginning I just kept running into Eric. I would see him at the same clothing stores, or we would see each other at the same recovery convention. Then we would come with an idea to throw our own Recovery Speaker Jam, or we would start up a new meeting together. Eric and I would see something that we liked, and we knew we could do something like that on our own. One weekend we went to a car show, and we decided to throw our own car show. We just kept things moving forward together rather than focusing on the past. Eventually we hosted some comedy shows together, which were a big hit. What I'm saying is, Eric is one of my go-to guys.

So, Eric, tell us something that you want to say to end all this. If there is one message you could put out there about recovery, this is your chance, man.

Eric: Yeah, one thing that I have learned throughout this process is, once you get into Narcotics Anonymous, you find out that recovery is not about the drugs. Recovery is about a disease that we have centered in our thinking. The way we see things, the way we relate to things, and the way we respond to things, that's where our addiction stems from. The game is a real disease, just like drug addiction. You just change the name, and you can put the same 12 steps on any problem that you got. The first three steps will always be significant. Admit that you have a problem. Once you admit or identify the problem, you figure out in step two what can help you with that problem. And once you figure out what can help you with that problem, you go to step three. Step three is allowing that help to help you. It's as simple as that. If you apply that process to anything you do, you'll come out with the answers. After those three steps, the fourth step is the key: step four is doing an inventory on yourself. When you do an inventory on the problem you are having, you'll find out what role you played in it, how you could have done it better, or what you would do different the next time. Once you figure all that out, you can't really worry about the other players because they have to do their own thing, but your side of the street is clean.

Richard: Well thank you, man, that was perfect. You made all that as clear as day, man. You hit all the necessary points. I really appreciate you taking the time to be a part of what I'm putting out for the people.

Eric: Absolutely, brother! I'll see you soon, and God bless.

CHAPTER 12

My Brother Kane

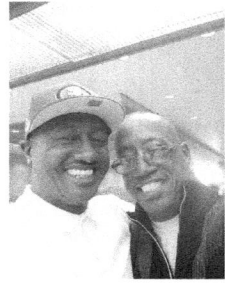

Larry and Richard

This is my older brother Larry, we grew up together in Richmond. Me and my brother have four sisters and four other brothers, so there are ten of us total. Four of the brothers are from the same mother and father, and the rest are kind of mixed around with other fathers and mothers. But Larry and I have the same father and mother. I was born is 1965, and Larry was born in 1963. The streets, and most of our family and friends, know my brother as Kane. I don't call him Kane; he's always been Larry or "Larry Lunch Meat" to me.

I used to get into a lot of trouble, a lot of fights, because I wore glasses and other kids gave me a hard time. Larry was always there for me, making sure I didn't get hurt. Our father would give us boxing gloves when me and my other brothers got into arguments, and we grew up boxing in our backyard back at the house. Larry was the best boxer out of all of us. Larry and I and our other two brothers were always getting into a lot of fights with the other kids in the neighborhood, because I talked a lot of shit.

Kane: Yeah, Ricky [Richard] was our baby brother, even though we have two brothers under us. We had a good life. We were never poor. And Ricky was always the baby boy. Our mom (Great Aunt) always used to say to me, "Larry, watch Ricky. You need to watch your baby brother." I took that assignment seriously.

Richard: Larry, talk about the P7 Hustlers, the hard times you had back in the day. Tell us who you are.

Kane: Growing up, our father Willie Bill never worked a traditional job a day in his life. Our father was a hustler, and he raised us to be self-sufficient and to be men. I remember my momma saying, "I can raise a boy, but I can't raise a man." Our mother sent us from 9th and Barret where we lived with her, to live with our father and let him raise us. When the government put all that powder, all that crack on the streets, me and my brothers were on those streets when all that took place. I didn't even know there was an age limit for drinking back when we were kids. I started drinking when I was thirteen years old, and that was nothing to anyone I was around. That was normal in our world.

I remember one night, way before Ricky got clean, Ricky and I were out in the streets hanging out, minding our business. This kid Anthony Mass tried taking something that was in Ricky's hand. Anthony was always bullying Richard, and Richard just could not take him. Anthony was bigger in every way than Richard, and I was just sick of seeing this go down, right. So that night I hit Anthony square in his mouth, not knowing that Anthony had a gun on him. We had to run for our lives. Another day, we were all at the Boys Club and here comes Anthony Mass, trying to bully Richard once again. We were all shooting pool or playing ping-pong when Anthony tried startin' some shit, and I was done with it. I was done with him messing with my little brother. I walked over to Anthony and I slapped him right across the face. Then me and my brothers shut down that entire area of the Boys Club because shit was about to go down. Once everything was shut down tight, I got on Anthony Mass, and I beat the ever-living hell out of that boy. I can remember yelling at Anthony, "You are not going to touch my little brother ever again!"

Richard: So what happened was, I wanted to fight Anthony Mass, but he got on top of me and started banging my head against the ground. After that is when Larry started calling me "Lump Lump," because my forehead had these two big-ass bumps from being slammed against the ground by Anthony Mass. When Larry saw that Anthony was wooping my ass, he ran over and kicked Anthony's ass. All I can remember is Larry pulling Anthony off of me, slapping Anthony across the face, then jumping on top of Anthony and using Anthony's face as a punching bag. But other kids said, "Larry is too big for Anthony. Let Richard fight Anthony again." So here I am fighting Anthony Mass again, my forehead is all lumped up, and then my other two brothers show up. All four of us Beal brothers chased Anthony Mass into another area of the Boys Club. We shut and locked the door behind us, and we started woopin' Anthony Mass with pool sticks.

Kane: We beat that boy down, man! And then we went outside. Somebody ended up calling the police, so the police are parked outside the Boys Club, all the kids from the Boys Club are outside, all just waiting for us. Remember, we were just children back then, but we weren't afraid to let everyone know that we were in charge and nobody was going to put a hand on any of us. I remember walking through all these people standing outside, and I walked right over to Anthony Mass and slapped the shit out of him one last time. I slapped that boy in front of the police, all those kids, and his entire family. I told that boy, "You are never putting your hands on my baby brother ever again, mother fucker!" I slapped that boy with my right hand so hard that I can still feel it to this day, man.

There was another family we used to call the "Bill Boys" back when we were in middle school. We used to have to catch the school bus, and the Bill Boys lived right outside where the bus picked us up. Well, the Bill Boys liked to mess with Richard because he wore glasses and because he was smaller than the rest of us. Our father had told us to put salt in our pockets, and he'd said when these boys tried to mess with us we should throw salt in their faces and start pounding on them. One morning we walked to that bus stop with salt in our pockets, and all the Bill Boys were waiting for us. Without giving it even a second thought, Richard threw that salt in one of those boy's eyes. I had never seen Richard fight like that before.

Richard: Damn right! Those guys were jealous of us because our father gave us all that weed to smoke and sell to the kids at our school. Our father was the weed man in our town, and some kids were jealous of that.

Kane: Our momma would always say, "Sticks and stones, words will never hurt me." But our father was like, "Nigga, you better get on that boy and show him who's in charge! Put some salt in your pocket and do what you gotta do." Man, I will never forget that morning. That was back when they first integrated us into a white neighborhood, and those Bill Boys thought they could take whatever they wanted from us because we were black. They weren't expecting us to woop their asses. Man, we went to work on those boys.

Richard: Back when we were in high school, Larry was one of the stars on the basketball team. The whole basketball team would come over to our house and smoke weed. We would go to the mini-market down the street, and a bunch of us would just grab everything we wanted and leave the store without paying. Fifteen of us would take as much as we could carry and run back home. We'd take the forty ouncers of Olde English, the chips, and premade sandwiches and just leave.

Kane: Everybody knew us. Everybody knew who our father was, and nobody wanted to mess with us. Nobody questioned us back then. I remember playing street ball at the 8th Street Park, and I used to knock them niggas out. Man, if you say something about my brother, I will beat your ass. I'd be playin' ball, I would dunk on your ass. You know, I was high school All American, McDonald's All American. I played for the Warriors for ten days back when Al Attles was the coach, and got paid $10,000. Man, back then we had the best athletes in the country in Richmond, California. My boy Dino, who played for the St. Louis Cardinals, lived right around the corner from us when we were kids.

Richard: Well, we knew him as Dino but his real name is Willie McGee. Willie McGee was MVP of the World Series.

Kane: Yeah, and I used to mess with Dino's sister. I'd go and see Dino after practice, and then the next thing you know, he was the MVP in the 1985 World Series. Dino was bow-legged and shy, but he could play some mother fuckin' ball, boy.

Richard: You went to prison, and you came out when my addiction really kicked off. When you first went in, I wasn't heavy on drugs yet. But when you got out, I was straight strung out, man.

Kane: Boy, when I got out of prison, my boy Richard was on one. Let me tell you a story about Lump Lump.

Richard: Ok, but before you go into anything, how much time did you do in prison?

Kane: If I were to add it all up, I have done about twenty-five years. But I did time in small increments. I'd do five years, then I'd do two years, then another five years. But all together, I have done twenty-five years. My longest stretch was seven years. And after that seven-year stretch, when I got out, you were on one, man.

Lump Lump used to sell BART tickets at the BART station, right. The day I got out, me and our father went to see Richard at the BART station. When we walked up to Richard, our father didn't even recognize him, he looked so bad. There was a time, if you threw a cigarette butt in a beer bottle, Richard would take that cigarette out of the beer bottle, drink whatever was left in the bottle, and wait for the cigarette to dry so he could smoke it. With my own two eyes I saw Richard do this.

Richard: This is true, but I had three or four good years of bein' "Dollar Bill" when you were in jail. But when you got out, I wasn't "Dollar Bill" anymore, I was "Twenty-Five Cents."

Kane: Let's talk about how you rose from all those hard times. Richard is my younger brother, but today Richard also is my hero. We lost our older brother, then we lost Bee-Bee. But Richard, he rose from the ashes. Every time I got out of prison I would come by St. Vincent DePaul, where he was working, and Richard would help me out with a little money. He would give me food. Growing up, Richard was always *Larry's brother*. But things flipped, and I became *Richard's brother*. Richard became the star of the family, and he helped me get to where I am at. Today Richard is runnin' shit. He's running the whole Tenderloin. I have three years clean, but Richard has thirty years clean, and he's the boss. I have seen my brother do some amazing things. Richard doesn't let anything or anyone get in the way of his recovery. In my eyes, Richard is invincible. And to work and live in the Tenderloin like my brother did for so many years, in the belly of the beast. For years I would say to Richard, "How are you doing this, man? How are you staying clean?"

Today I work on 8th and Market. I take my lunch to work, because I don't want to even walk around the TL and get tempted by what is going on over there. I used to walk to Richard's office, and he would be wearing his big hats and his furs and shiny shoes and carrying his gold cane. Richard inspires me today. I get lazy sometimes, but all I have to do is think about my brother Richard and then I get up and go about my day. Richard bought his first house recently. Nobody else in our family has actually owned their own home.

Richard: You said that Pops never worked. We never saw our father go to a 9-to-5 job. He just hustled til the day he died.

Kane: I believe that was instilled into all of us. I used to rob banks, grocery stores. I used to rob other drug dealers, I used to rob jewelry stores, you name it, man. I can't blame our father for the wrongs that I did, but our father did show us how to get down. The first time I went to Folsom Prison it was for robbing a bank—man, I threw so much of my life away back then. I had my daughter, London, I was a star athlete, and here I was robbing banks in order to get my kicks. On one side I was bringing home trophies, and on the other side I was bringing home bags of stolen money. I remember one day I brought home this one basketball trophy for being the year's highest scorer, but my dad was mad at me because there were so many dirty dishes in the sink. He took the trophy out of my hand, threw it, and told me to clean all those dishes in the sink. Our father would always tell us, "I'm not your friend, I'm your father."

Richard: Our father didn't mess around. If you weren't bringing home money, our father didn't care.

Kane: Yeah, I remember Richard used to stay at one of our father's gambling houses. What street was that on?

Richard: We moved the gambling between different houses, but I stayed at one of the houses that hosted gambling parties. We didn't want anyone to know exactly where the gambling was happening. A guy named Lincoln had a house, a guy named Banks had a house, and then there was Stan Hill and our father. So, between those four houses they rotated who would host the gambling parties. Moving the gambling parties around made it next to impossible for any one of us to get robbed. Sometimes they would move the party to another house at the last minute.

On one occasion, one of our father's friends ran out of money, but he wanted to keep gambling and he refused to leave. Our father told the guy that he needed to leave, and the guy said, "What are you going to do, Willie Bill? You ain't goin' to do nothing, Willie Bill!" Our father hit him with a short right hand, and knocked that guy out. And then Larry started going through that guy's pockets.

Kane: I missed a lot because I was in prison, but I remember those moments. When I got out, me and my brother Bee-Bee got close. Bee-Bee and I were less than nine months apart, and Bee-Bee was my nigga. Me and Bee-Bee used to hang out a lot in the TL. Bee-Bee used to cut hair, and we would just shoot the shit for hours and hours.

Richard: When I got clean, Larry and Bee-Bee used to wreak havoc on the Tenderloin. Every time they got into trouble they would drop my name. "Oh, I'm Richard's brother. Just call Richard and he'll tell you who I am." Every time something went down, I would get a call.

Kane: As children growing up, I saw my brother rise. In the belly of the beast, I saw him rise. I just have to keep saying this because it was a miracle. Richard likes to showboat, he's flamboyant, and he is who he is going to be, but it is 100% real. Thanks to Richard, I have two degrees, I don't know how many certificates I have, I have traveled all over the world, and it's all because of my brother Richard. We have shaken the hands of multiple presidents, we hang out with mayors, and people listen to us. I have been able to change all my old ways because I saw Richard change his old ways. I don't think I could have done all that without him.

Richard: Larry, if you wanted to say one thing about this project we are working on, how *we* recovered from the game, how *we* survived, what would you say to people coming out of the game right now?

Kane: You know, you can talk til your head falls off. It's not about what you say. It's you. You have to be tired and done with all the bad shit you are doing. You can't have any more energy left for all that mess. I live in a nice little spot in Oakland right now, but every day I see all the grime we have been talking about. But the only thing that can change an individual is the individual himself. I can tell someone exactly what I did. I can tell them what meetings I went to and who I talked to and learned from, but it would all be for nothing if the person I was talking to wasn't ready to change. Change always has to be up to you. When you say, "I'm done! I'm tired!" and you really mean those words, then you can change. But if you don't really mean it, you won't change. You have to be done, and you have to be resilient.

You know, our father passed away when he was sixty-one. Our oldest brother, Anthony, passed away when he was fifty-five. And that right there motivates me. I just turned sixty-one, and I want to live a long and healthy life. And if our father was still alive today and you were to look at our father, you'd see me and Richard. We look just like our father. In order for me to keep goin' and live a long life, I have to keep changing my ways. I can't blame society, it's not the white man or that I was raised to be a certain way. No, it's up to the individual to change.

CHAPTER 13

Del from the TL

Del and I do a lot of events together. We do Recovery Day, we speak at different recovery platforms throughout the country, we organize rallies we support each other as much as we can. I work for Tenderloin Housing Clinic and Del is the founder of Code Tenderloin. Del is actually the founder of everything that has to do with recovery in the Tenderloin Neighborhood. Everybody calls Del "the Mayor of the Tenderloin" and everybody calls me "the Ambassador of the Tenderloin." We just go together. And I feel blessed that I am able to bring Del into this book, because I want everyone to know who Del is. Let's get down to business here. I want to introduce you all to my good friend, Del Seymour.

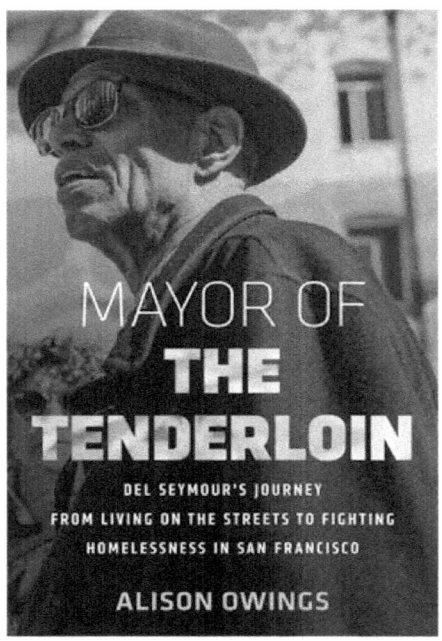

Del from the TL

Del: I grew up in Chicago and went into the service during the Vietnam War. When I got out of the service, I didn't want to go back to Chicago because it's too cold. I'd gotten used to warm weather during the war, so I decided to go to LA. While I was in LA, I became a fire fighter and a paramedic, and I had kids. Eventually my kids moved to the Bay Area, and I decided to follow them up since I was coming up every weekend to see them. That's how I met the Tenderloin. I didn't even know what the Tenderloin was, but after being in the neighborhood for about eight hours, I *became* the Tenderloin. I didn't realize how deep I got into my addiction the first day of being here. I became a full-blown addict that first day. I don't even know what year this was. I stopped keeping track of years and dates a long time ago. I don't "stir." You know, I tell people all the time, don't let no one ask you when or where something happened, because you are just stirring that memory. You don't need to bother that memory. Leave that shit alone! Man, you can say, well one day I got started. You can say, well see, what day was that? Who was I with? What did I buy? How did it hit me? That's stirring that pot. I don't stir the pot, brother. And I don't count days, man. Well, how many years? I don't know man, it's been about fourteen, fifteen, sixteen years. I don't have no anniversary date. 'Cause again, that's like counting like it's going to stop. My sobriety off drugs ain't never going to stop. So why in the hell would I be I counting?

You know, there are different disciplines in recovery. This is the discipline that I find works out for me. It may not work out for you. It may not work out for anyone else, but it works well for me. And that's how we have to do this thing. We got to find our own path. We can get guidance from all the recovery groups and our mentors and our sponsors and all our fellow people in recovery, but at the end of the day, it has to be something that affects you. 'Cause you got your addiction on your own, so you need to get your recovery on your own as far as what hits you right.

I personally go to several recovery groups a week, and all the people that I know are very flexible. We don't get down on nobody for whatever they do or what they say, their method, or anything like that. Some of their methods I think are crazy as hell. But I've been in these groups for years with the same people, and they're keepin' their sobriety up with their crazy-ass method. I should say that, just because *I* think it's crazy doesn't mean it *is* crazy. If what you are doing works, keep doin' it. I don't knock anyone for doing anything, including harm reduction. Who the hell am I? They could be in the worst situation that they could possibly be in, and they might be hittin' something once a week. Or they could be hittin' it every day, whatever "it" is, right. I'm not going to knock them for that. I would like to see one day when they don't hit that pipe at all. But if they're coming to the meetings and sharing their stories, you can't knock that, man. It is very important to me that I get out that message that there are a lot of people out there tryin' to get clean, trying to improve their lives. Everybody has a different path and time frame when it comes to living their lives.

I was out there living the life of an addict for eighteen years, give or take. I was a drug dealer. I was the biggest dealer on Turk and Taylor. I also was the biggest drug user on Turk and Taylor. I got shot, got stabbed, went to jail four times. I was lookin' at my rap sheet this morning. Fourteen felonies on Turk and Taylor for drug sales. I lived a far-out life for a long time. I was finally able to get clean from those drugs and those demons. I got clean through my children, through my church, through watching other people, and through just being tired. A lot of people will say, "Oh, you'll stop when you get sick and tired." No, no, you need more than that, 'cause I was sick and tired for seventeen or eighteen years and I didn't stop. Once I got around people that were clean, and once I got used to being around those people, I started to notice that I liked that new kind of relationship. I liked those sober people. They were honest, they really cared for me, they had no motives, and that was a brand-new world for me. Because when you're in a drug scenario, everybody's got a motive. Your girl, your dude, your neighbor, the dude at the grocery store, everybody's got a motive because they know you're a dope fiend. Ain't nobody goin' to give you nothin' when you're a dope fiend unless they can get something back. So, I got around people who weren't like that, and in the beginning I was skeptical. "Why are you giving me this? What do you want from me?" When I was first starting out in recovery, a lady gave me $100. A few days later I got some money so I tried to pay that lady back, but she said, "No, that was not a loan. That was a gift. I am Christian and we don't lend money." It took me a long time to understand the concept of unconditional love. Love without motive. I started to run into more and more people who had no motives. "Oh, you can come and crash at my house tonight." And? "No, just come and crash out at my house tonight." I would go over there with a lot of suspicion in the back of my mind and find that there was nothing but love.

When I first got sober and started going to church, I was still homeless. People would invite me to spend the night at their house so I had a safe place to be. These people would go to Macy's that same day and buy me clothes. No motives! I couldn't wrap my mind around this in the beginning, but this became a new model for my life. I wanted to be the type of man that helped people and didn't expect anything back. No motives. That is a major part of recovery: we start doing things for people without expecting any kind of payment. Not in front of the camera. Not in front of the spotlights. Just on the under. Give somebody some money on the under. Don't tell nobody else you did it. When you tell somebody you did something good, that's a motive. I'm not a Bible person at all, but I think somewhere in the Bible it says that's how a giver is supposed to be. This is the kind of man I am today, and it's a very rewarding way to live your life.

I was in Chicago not too long ago, and I had to go to a UPS store to take care of some business. Right outside the front door of the UPS store was this woman who was in pretty rough shape. I could tell right away that this woman was a crack user, but you know, I don't down nobody for what they do. 'Cause I was her years ago, right. This woman stops me and says, "Hey man, can I get a few dollars? I'm hungry and I haven't eaten in two days." I went in my pocket and all I had was a $10 bill, so I gave it to her. As I went into the UPS store, in the back of my mind I just assumed that woman was going to go buy $10 worth of crack, no big deal, right. I was in the UPS store for about ten minutes, then I came out of the store and I was getting into my car. In that same parking lot was a Wendy's, and here she comes out of the Wendy's with a drink and a bag of food. It touched my heart that I misjudged her, and you can't do that with people. I don't want to judge people like that. You know, you take a risk sometimes, helping someone, but so what? People took a risk on us, and we burned them. As a drug addict, we burn a lot of people. And that's part of life. So, why can't I take a chance on someone? When did I become too good for that? I remember seeing that woman come out of Wendy's with that big bag of food, and it moved me to tears. I misjudged that woman and it crushed me.

As my recovery goes on, I learn more about myself. Recovery can take place in so many different ways. Recovery can mean you stop smoking. But if you're still jumping over the BART gates, that's not recovery. Yeah, you stopped smoking, but you're still going to Safeway and putting stuff in your pocket. You're still lying to your baby momma about not having enough money for child support, but you don't smoke no more. I'm sorry to tell you, but you're not in recovery, bro. My thing in recovery is to get better than what you were. To restore all your principles. A person in recovery becomes a typical person: you don't steal, you don't lie, you don't cheat, you don't jump over the BART gate. Even though nobody is sitting at the station, you just pay your ticket. That's when you know you're in recovery. If you go in the store and the lady gives you too much change back, you give that money back to her. That's my idea of maintaining recovery. It's to get my life together, to get my house in order. I keep my house immaculate, and part of that is not just recovery but from my military training. When I leave my home it looks like a model house, even if I'm going to be gone for an hour. My house is clean. That's part of my recovery. I wash my car every other day. That's part of my recovery. Clean mind, clean body, clean car, clean house. All of that, man. You got to dress different from those old days.

I was walking in the Tenderloin in one of my three-piece suits the other day, and I saw one of the guys that I used to use with twenty years ago. He was layin' on the sidewalk, and he looked at me and he said, "Del, you think you're better than everyone else." I said, "I'm better than you, bro, because I ain't smokin' that shit no more. Yes, I am better than everyone else that's smoking that shit. And I want you to be the same way." So, yeah, I am not you, and I *am* better than you. That's the attitude that we have to have if we are going to make it in recovery. Just now, a guy a block and half from here stopped me and introduced himself to me. And I said, "Yeah man, it's nice to meet you." And he says to me, "No, we met years ago. And I've watched you, and man, I have tried to model my life after the things that you do." You don't know how many people come up to me and say that. It's important for us in recovery to be that model for others. It's important that we talk, right. It's important that we make time for people. We have to take the time and listen to people. There are days when I'm walking in the Tenderloin and it takes me one hour to walk a block because people want to talk. People want to be heard, and most other people don't want to listen to them. I'll listen. I have to listen. That's part of it, man. That's part of being a recovery leader in this community of the Tenderloin. Back in the day I helped break things, so today I am helping fix things. I want to make things right. And there aren't a whole bunch of us out here. A lot of people are in recovery in the TL, but they haven't got to the level that Richard and I are at. It's our job to help the people that want to be where we are get there, right. That's our job. And some people in recovery just have to be who they are, right. And that's cool. It's not a requirement to be me or Richard. But if you want to get to where Richard and I are at, we'll help you. That's why I started Code Tenderloin. To give people in the Tenderloin a chance to get off the ground. To get a better position in life. Jobs, housing, connecting people together. That's what Code Tenderloin does, and we don't charge a penny.

Richard: Code Tenderloin runs the Ambassador Program and job training programs. And Del also does his walking tours.

Del: Yeah, I've been doing walking tours of the Tenderloin for eighteen years. And in those eighteen years I think I've walked 85,000 people around the TL. The point of the walking tours is to give people who don't live in the Tenderloin the opportunity to see the better parts of this neighborhood. I stop by art galleries, cafes, restaurants, and a bunch of other places, and I'll talk with people like Richard who have great stories to tell. I am so proud to know people like Richard. I am proud to be involved with Richard. We can all depend on Richard to take care of the people we bring to him to be taken care of. We know that all the people we send to Richard will be treated fairly, and we know that Richard will not have any outside motives. Richard just wants to help.

Code Tenderloin has our Night Navigators, who walk around the TL until four in the morning. We are dealing with harm reduction facilities. We help people get medications that can soothe their addiction until we can get them into a treatment facility.

Richard: Del was right there for our fourth annual Recovery Day, and we're getting ready to do the fifth one in 2025. Del was right there when Mayor Breed gave me an award for all my work with the Recovery Community in the Tenderloin. Del always brings his entire team from Code Tenderloin to help plan our Recovery Day events every year. Del has become one of my mentors over the years, and I have learned so much from him. Del tells his story in the 2024 memoir, *Mayor of the Tenderloin: Del Seymour's Journey from Living on the Streets to Fighting Homelessness in San Francisco*, which I bought the moment it came out.

Del comes from Chicago and I come from Richmond, but we both came here to San Francisco's Tenderloin neighborhood. When I came out here to San Francisco, I was following the dope. Everyone told me that you could smoke all the dope you want in San Francisco and not get arrested. Back in the day that sounded like heaven to me, so I came right on down to the Tenderloin.

Del: Same here! Once I found out what the Tenderloin was and that there were no consequences for doing the amount of drugs I wanted to do, I was sold.

Everybody ends up at the Tenderloin. But here we are now, years later, clean, trying to repair some of the damage that we created. Because we did do a lot of damage out here. We sold a lot of drugs out here. We did a lot of drugs out here. We robbed people, we broke into buildings, and we did whatever we had to do to get our dope or sell our dope to get more dope. I used a lot of drugs in Boeddeker Park. So it is amazing that we turned that park, which was a drug den for so many years, into sanctuary for people to feel safe. Boeddeker Park has become a sanctuary for recovery. Children play there, we have events there, and it's part of the heart of the Tenderloin now. People tell me, "Oh man, Recovery Day is getting too big. You have to move away from Boeddeker Park," but I tell them, "I'm not ever moving from Boeddeker Park." Now, if they want to start something somewhere else in the city they can, but there ain't no Recovery Day like the Recovery Day at Boeddeker Park. That's because of what that park once was and what it is today.

Del: You are exactly right, yeah.

Richard: Del, if you have any last words that you want our readers to hear before you sign off, now is the time to do it.

Del: Well, you know, I wanted to use every day for about three years when I first got clean. When I first got sober and I was giving my tours in the TL in those early days, some of those voices telling me to get high would come back into my head, and when that happened, I immediately ran over to the BART station. I would leave everyone on the tour, and I'd get out of town. So I moved out of San Francisco for a bit, and I went out to Fairfield, California. I just couldn't fight my demons in the Tenderloin. I needed to get out so I could get comfortable with the new me. I needed to get some of the edge off. After about a year I felt comfortable enough to move back to the city. So I think if I could say anything to someone that is new to recovery, I would just say, do what you have to do. Whatever is going to help you stay clean, just do that. There is no magic password that will help everyone. We are all different, and we all need slightly different things to help us.

CHAPTER 14

From the Queen's Perspective

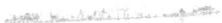

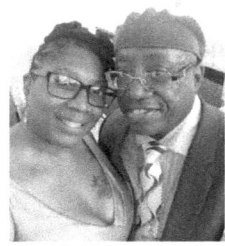

The Queen and me

I can't really see myself completing this book project without having the love of my life, my queen, in this. And whether she knows it or not, my wife LaTonya Crystal Kelly Beal, has been the backbone of my recovery. When I get home from work, my wife is the person I rely on for ease and comfort. It is only right to have my wife's perspective seeing the progression of my recovery over the last seven years. In October 2024 we just celebrated seven years of marriage. And January 8,' 2025, we celebrated eight years since our first date. LaTonya was there when I decided to bring Recovery Day back to life. She was the person I called when my brother died, and she came over and cleaned him up before the paramedics showed up. I want to make this introduction short and sweet so LaTonya can have her moment. So here she is, Mrs. LaTonya Crystal Kelly Beal.

LaTonya: Growing up, I had been around a few people that had the disease of addiction. I had seen my aunt struggle a bit. On occasion, family members would talk about my aunt always needing money, or borrowing things and never returning them. She would lose a lot of weight and then gain it back during those times when she would try to clean herself up for appearance's sake. Eventually my aunt always went back to her bad behavior. Overall, I lived a fairly sheltered life in East Oakland. I remember going on East 14th Street, which is now International Boulevard, and my parents would tell me to be careful. My fathered owned a grocery store, and after school I would walk to his store, but my parents would always remind me to be careful of the people walking around. My parents always told me to stay away from drugs. I remember when a man named Felix Mitchell, who was a well-known drug dealer in Oakland, passed away, and there was this big funeral for him. The funeral was on TV, and everyone wore white suits and dresses, and there was even a horse-drawn carriage. It really seemed like Felix Mitchell was this local superstar. My mother was frustrated because Felix brought a lot of drugs into our community for a long time, and she couldn't understand why people would want to lift him up, as if he had done good for the city of Oakland.

My parents had a large wine collection in our basement and would drink wine with dinner, but that was the extent of alcohol use in my household. I never saw anyone get drunk at my house, not even at family parties. Losing control was something my family just never did. There was always a sense of balance and control under our roof. But when I was twenty-two years old, I got married to a man who I later realized was an alcoholic. There were no signs that my husband had a drinking problem while we were dating. There were no red flags for me to see. I would say it was about four years into our marriage that my husband's alcoholism started to take over. I started finding bottles all over the house. Sometimes he would urinate in the closet because he didn't know where he was. He started blacking out more and more. At this time, I was in college for a bachelor's degree in human services, and I started taking this class on chemical dependency. I wanted to understand what was going on with my husband. Through that class I started to understand that my husband had a disease, and it was much more serious than I was aware of. That class helped me grow to have compassion for my husband and all people with the disease of addiction. Once I started to understand more about my husband's disease, I started telling him that there were meetings he could go to for his disease. I would tell him that he could get help and he didn't have to go through all this on his own. I was there for him, but I knew he needed a community in order to really get better. After a while of trying to get my husband to find help, I had to acknowledge that he didn't really want help, so we ended up separating.

As my career went on as a Mental Health Rehabilitation Specialist, I would come across clients who not only had a mental illness but also had some kind of chemical dependency disorder at the same time. I saw how this was really challenging for them, and I developed another level of compassion for my clients. Around this time, I met Richard. I actually met Richard while I was on vacation from work. I had some extra time on my hands, and someone from the church where I used to co-pastor called me and asked me to go pray and sit with a woman in need. That woman turned out to be Richard's stepmom. I spent some time with Richard's stepmom, and as I was about to leave her house, Richard dropped by and we got to talking a bit. After our first conversation, Richard asked if he could see me again, and I agreed.

The one thing that really struck me about Richard is that he immediately told me about these 12-step meetings he was committed to attending. He let me know right away that recovery was his number one thing in life, but he really wanted to get to know me. I used to go to some of the meetings with Richard. I went partially out of personal interest in the world that he was a part of, but I also went simply because I wanted to support Richard. I loved what he had to say in his shares. I would go to Speaker Jams with Richard on occasion, and I was just blown away by some of the things that I heard. I was being introduced into a whole other world. I felt like I had an inside view of this thing that I had only seen on TV or read about in the newspaper. Hearing so many people's stories was an incredible experience for me, and to hear Richard's story was especially incredible. The first time I heard Richard's story, I was like, "Wow! This man is a miracle."

I would cry sometimes because I was overwhelmed with how so many people had found a way to overcome their demons. I just call it the Holy Spirit. What else can explain how some of these people were able to survive the things they went through and come out the other end, not only in one piece but even better than when they started? How does someone put themself back together without a higher power? How does someone learn to love themself again? I had never seen men, especially black men, hug each other and tell each other that they loved each other before. I had never seen black men be so vulnerable with each other before. I didn't even know that existed, to be honest with you. There was so much love in those rooms that Richard took me to. I loved being in the middle of the energy of those spaces, and I loved being able to stand next to Richard while all this positivity was happening. I have always supported Richard and his work that he does.

Another thing that really blew me away was this whole thing about service. You can see how people behave at the meetings, but you never know what those people are like when they are outside of the meetings. You don't get to see how people treat each other when they get home. But I got to see how Richard applied the steps of the program outside of the meetings. I got to see how Richard applied the steps while he was at home and in his personal life. I got to see how Richard applied the steps in our life together. I have been able to witness firsthand Richard's discipline, and the sense of integrity that he has. This made me love Richard even more, because I saw how he was sincere in what he was doing. Richard didn't just talk about how important service was, he really embodied service in all aspects of his life, and he still does to this day. I really admire the way that Richard shows up for life, and when I think about this it makes me want to support him even more.

After Richard gave me a deep look into his work, I wanted to be closer to the people in the rooms and the world of recovery. There was a rawness to everything I was seeing and everyone I was meeting, and I wanted to be closer to that. I value authenticity and the people Richard surrounds himself with embody what I want to surround myself with.

Richard: Could you talk a little bit about Recovery Day? How you learned to interact with people at that event and at other events like Recovery Day that we have attended together?

LaTonya: In the beginning of Richard's and my marriage, I met up with him at his office. I remember catching BART, getting off on Market Street, and walking through the Tenderloin in order to get to Richard's office. This sense of culture shock come over me, because I had never spent any time in the Tenderloin before. All the drugs, people sleeping or passed out on the sidewalks, all the different smells. The Tenderloin District is probably overwhelming to anyone the first time they walk through it. It was for me. I had never seen someone shoot up on the street before. I remember Richard was walking me back to the BART station, and this guy came up to us and he was like, "Hey, Richard, do you remember when you were out here on the street with us?" And that's when it really hit home for me. I had heard Richard's story, and over time I would get to learn more about Richard's past. But I didn't know all the details of his past at that particular time, and it had never really hit me what it meant to be homeless until I saw all those people in the TL for the first time. The good thing that I took from that day is my understanding that if Richard was able to get sober and get off the streets, then other people could do it as well. I knew there was hope for *all* those people. If someone with the disease of addiction chooses to get help, they will have a chance at a better life.

I believe that it is a miracle when someone decides to get help, that a higher power is present at that moment. I believe that we all have access to a higher power. I bring up that day because that experience helped me to see what events like Recovery Day are all about. I started to realize that there is a whole spectrum of people and experiences that people are living right now. All the people from different backgrounds coming together for a common goal is a beautiful thing.

After spending the last seven years with Richard and watching the work that he does, I started thinking that Richard and I could merge what we do and help both our communities together. We recently took over a space on the corner of 6th and Stevenson in San Francisco, and we are in the phase of putting our heads together to figure out what we want to do there. I am not sure yet how we will activate this space and integrate it into the community.

There is a reality that comes with its location that I still have to wrap my mind around. Just the other day I was parked right outside our new space, sitting in the passenger seat, and people pulled up right by my car with their drug paraphernalia and they started using right next to my car. I couldn't even open my door to get out, and that freaks me out, to be perfectly honest with you. It makes me sad to see that level of poverty. But I still do my best to see them in the highest light possible and to see the humanity in everyone. Sixth Street is a harsh environment, and it's something that I'm not used to nor do I want to see, but I know these people need help. Some of them might actually want the help we can give them. I feel that if we find the right way to go about activating our new space, we can use it to help people. I want to fight for my ideas and fight for the people that I see using drugs on the streets of San Francisco. I want to provide a space for people to thrive. I want people to have a place where they feel safe, and they can be their authentic self. I want people to find not only themselves but to find other people who are on a similar journey, and create a new community. This is a humanitarian project in my mind. I want to address the loneliness and disconnection that so many of us feel on a daily basis. I want to meet people where they are, but I don't want to leave them that way. I would like to have the time to sit down with someone, find out what their individual needs are, and help them find what they are looking for. If we come across someone with needs we are not able to meet, we can do some research for them and point them in the right direction rather than just leave them out in the cold. I would like our space to serve multiple functions. I would like to provide a home base for people, or to act as a bridge that will lead someone to the place they should be.

I have worked as a case manager, a social worker, and a program director for many years, and one thing I have noticed is that a lot of our current spaces, especially our institutionalized spaces, have not been able to look at a person as a whole. These larger organizations that are trying to help the homeless, mentally ill individuals, and people suffering with addiction are not able to offer holistic approaches. And because of this, a lot of things get missed when trying to treat someone. I think some of these organizations might be so big that they are not able to take the time to really get to know their clients. There are so many patients and only so much time in a day to treat them, and when you are always in a rush and running on fumes, people are going to fall through the cracks. I want to help those people that fall through society's cracks. I want the people I work with to feel seen and heard.

The more I think about it, I really want to turn the nonprofit model into more of a non-religious faith-based space. I want to operate more like a covert temple of some kind, without calling it a temple because that has its own connotation. We talk about all these different types of services that we want to provide, but where can the people gather and just be? Where can these people go to decompress from all the stresses of the street and street life? Where can these people go to experience culture, to have some fun, to think things through, to talk things out with another person who cares? I want our space to not only provide resources but to also have an information desk to share about other resources that the city has to offer as well.

Richard: The guy that we rent the new space over on 6th Street from is Dipak Patel, who also owns this building, the Drake Hotel. I would never have been able to do Recovery Day without Dipak. Every time I call Dipak for something, he always delivers. Dipak gave us a donation of $3,000 for our last Recovery Day event. His family owns small hotels all over the city of San Francisco through their company, RPM Management. His family also owns the 200-room Seneca Hotel, right next door to the building space that we are leasing. The company I work for, the Tenderloin Housing Clinic, has been managing the Seneca Hotel for RPM Management since 1995. The Seneca Hotel and our new space are in the heart of the 6th Street corridor, an area with a lot of history. We are about to begin a whole new journey, and I assure you it is going to be a wild ride. The space we just took over actually was a skate shop for years, and when the skate shop left the space just sat empty for a while. It's in the heart of the area where we need to be, and the space needs to be filled.

LaTonya: I intend to lift up the people who lift up the people. One of the things that we see in the case management and social work fields is high burnout, compassion fatigue, and high turnover. I want our space to be multi-use, so the support and help we offer also includes the people who are helping those in the most need. Those staff members who work in all those facilities all over the city of San Francisco also need help and services. Whether that be sound healing, mindfulness, meditation, reiki sessions, or just someone to talk to, I want to provide these services. When people come through our doors, their titles and roles don't matter because everyone is coming into this community to receive love and to receive whatever class or event is going on. I think we all deserve to just chill out if we want to, right. I see it as a place that can support practitioners who may have a small business, or work at a large hospital, or maybe they provide some kind of service on their own and they are always on the go. They can come in and receive services the same way that a resident or a client of one of these transitional houses in the Tenderloin can come in.

Recently Richard saw this article about a program where someone could go to a ballet class and receive the same credit as going to a meeting or another means of treating their addiction. When I was talking to Richard about this I was like, "Yeah, that makes sense. Why can't an activity like ballet support your recovery?" Exercise is good for you regardless of the type of exercise you are getting. I believe there are many ways to heal and recover. I can't speak from the same perspective as someone who is in recovery from the disease of addiction, but I can speak on how important it is for someone to be in one's body and have a relationship with the body I am in, my body. I can speak on how important it is to respect oneself and love oneself. I understand how important it is to be able to de-stress mentally and physically, and to remove trauma from one's body. Movement is key to the process of someone feeling better about themself. Movement is important to healing from the inside out. I want to provide a space that allows people to build bridges between their mental, physical, and spiritual self. I think being able to go to one place where you can meditate, take a yoga class or a ballet class, maybe be part of a podcast, or just sit down and talk to someone about your troubles would be an amazing thing, and this is what I intend to do.

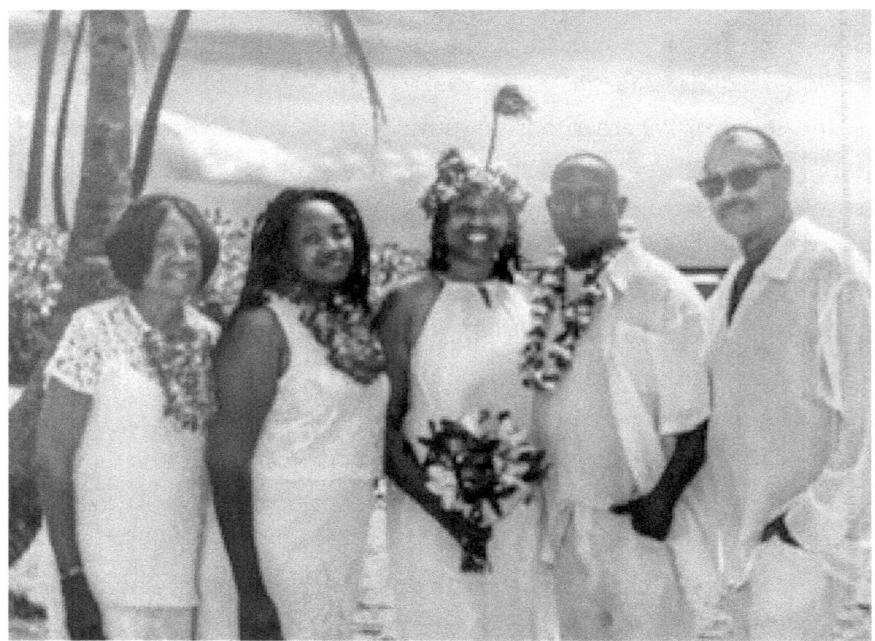

Our wedding party in Hawaii

My final thought on this is, back when I was taking those classes on chemical dependency, all the books told me that only 5% people who seek out recovery and long-term abstinence from drugs and alcohol make it. I don't know where these people that write these books get their information, but if 5% is the real number, that information was always profound to me. That 5% was one of the things that I carried into the rooms with me back when I was checking out NA meetings. Seeing the recovery in the rooms that I went to really blew me away. The only question I have ever had is, how can we increase that 5% success rate? What will it take? And I think the way to address that number is by addressing the whole person. I can only do my small part. I can offer love, and I can listen. We can take that space on 6th Street and turn it into something special with the help of other like-minded people. Let's just pour as much love and good intention into it as possible, so that it can ripple out into the community and the city of San Francisco.

Richard: This has been fantastic! I want to thank you, my wife, my queen. Thank you for being in my life. You are the best part of me, and I couldn't create a book about recovering from anything without you being a part of it. I so appreciate you taking time out to be part of this project.

CHAPTER 15

Epilogue

You know, I look forward for this book to get out there because I just don't believe that the game is "to be sold and not told." I think that we have to tell what the game was about. And today, to me, "GAME" stands for Good Advice Means Everything. People have heard me say that a million times over the years. That's a Richard Beal quote right there. I'm excited about turning sixty years old this year with thirty years clean. I'm thinking about celebrating my thirty years with all my loved ones. Thirty years of doing service in recovery. I can't say it enough: I am grateful, man. You know when they say, "Lost dreams awaken, new possibilities arise." That's me. I was like the phoenix rising out of the ashes thirty years ago. I'm that caterpillar that turned into a butterfly. I didn't give up. I come from that No Matter What school. Don't take nothin', no matter what. My mother died, my father died, my brothers died, I watched my second wife take her last breath, I got phone calls about other people passing away, and I didn't take nothin'.

But as we know, the disease can manifest itself in different ways. I got caught up in gambling, but my last bet was on October 31, 2022. After a wake-up call, I found myself in Gamblers Anonymous. A good friend told me that I really needed to check out GA and get my mind straight, because I was on the road to causing myself some real financial problems if I didn't get myself straightened out. So that's what I did. And working Gamblers Anonymous taught me that I can't discriminate where I get my help from. I mean, right now, I am sitting at my desk and I have my GA book right here. I've got my *Just for Today* book, I've got my *One Day at a Time* book, I've got *Living Clean*, I've got *Daily Reflections*, I've got Cocaine Anonymous and Alcoholics Anonymous books right over here. I've got all my books right here, man. I am open to it all and I need it all. The disease of addiction is all over the place for me, man. And I have enough freedom in my recovery so I can walk into any 12-step meeting and respect the traditions of whatever that fellowship is. You know, it's all good, man.

I walked into an AA meeting in the '80s, before I was clean. I was trying to get clean, but I wasn't ready yet. I started talking about crack and dope, but people would cut me off and tell me they don't talk about drugs in AA. But things are a lot different today. Today, in most AA meetings, you can talk about most anything you want as long as it's about recovery. But back in the '80s, things were a lot tighter, which was discouraging for me. Today I can walk into AA and everyone embraces me and my story. Nobody shuts me down today. In my mind, addiction is addiction, and alcohol is just one symptom of the disease of addiction. When I talk about the disease of addiction, I am talking about sex addition, food addiction, gambling, cocaine, alcohol, pornography; whatever kind of addiction is out there, there is a group for you to go to. If you need to go to OA, FA, CA, ACA, NA, AA, all of that, find what works for you so you don't end up with the "ME," the Medical Examiner. If you don't do anything about your disease, you are going to end up with the "ME," and somebody is going to pick you up in a body bag.

I am so blessed to have a completely different outlook on my addiction and my life as a whole today. The outlook I have today allows me to work with organizations like the Department of Public Health. I was lucky enough to be instrumental in organizing the first Overdose Prevention Summit, held on January 30, 2025, at the San Francisco Public Library. I have been able to be part of the San Francisco Recovery Coalition. Recently we did a rally and a march from Downtown all the way to the steps of City Hall. We spoke with San Francisco's City Supervisors Dorsey, Stefani, Mandelman, and Safai. We talked about a program called "Read to Recover," where you can go to the San Francisco Public Library and take home a recovery-based book to keep, for free. Whether it's the AA Big Book, the NA Big Book, a recovery-based book written by a sober author, you can keep that book. That right there is helping addicts who want to get clean. I have been able to do some speaking engagements with the organization "Mothers Against Drug Overdoses." My good friend Del Seymour, "The Mayor of the Tenderloin," and I do a lot of work together. When Del finished his book, he held a book signing at this place called Manny's over on 16th and Valencia, and I was right there in the front row supporting Del.

I think about what this is all about. My past life. That battle with addiction. Recovery and helping people with their battle and their personal tug of war between their disease and their recovery. I am on a mission today. I truly believe that the God of my understanding has given me an assignment. He has assigned me to carry the good news: *Recovery is possible!* You can recover from homelessness. No matter where you come from, it doesn't matter. The only thing that matters is where you want to go and what you want to do with your life. My God has empowered me to instill hope in others. And that's heavy, man.

All of the people mentioned in this book were role models for me. I don't believe that people die so I can live, I believe that some people lived so that I wouldn't die. If it weren't for those predecessors and people that embraced me, I know I wouldn't be here today. I have had so many moments in the spotlight because of these people, but today I don't want to be in the spotlight. I want to be the light in the spot. I want to shine the light of God and show you what the God of my understanding has done for me. If God could do it for me, he could do it for anybody else. That's what all this is about. And the God of *your* understanding could be Good Orderly Direction, it could be the Great Out Doors, it could be Group of Dope fiends, but it can't be *you*. It can't be just you, man! Hope comes from hearing other people's experiences. And hope stands for Hold On Pain Ends, and Happy Our Program Exists.

You know, I can't close out without saying that I think we need drug-free housing. The ideal environment for an addict coming out of treatment or jail would be to go into drug-free supportive housing. Drug-free supportive housing needs to have integrated services, such as behavioral health services and medical health professionals on-site. The ideal environment should have units with panic buttons that you can push if someone is overdosing or having a heart attack or some other kind of medical emergency. Things like that are a better use of our funding than giving people free pipes, tin foil, and Brillo pads. I understand the concept of harm reduction, but if I just got clean yesterday, the last thing you should be giving me is a free pipe, tin foil, and a Brillo pad. I don't think I would have been able to stay clean if I was given that stuff. *You are going to give me a brand-new crack pipe every day? Ok, let's go!* That's what my addict brain is going to tell me. So I thank God that I got clean when I did, man. I am drug free, but I'm not drug proof. I understand that, and that's why I continue to go to meetings. When I hear that people relapsed, I always hear the same thing: they got disconnected, they stopped going to meetings, they stopped hanging around people who are in recovery, they decided to take full control over their life, they listened to their own BS, and they got loaded. I truly believe that my mind is unsafe territory. *Do not go inside without adult supervision.* It has been declared by many as a weapon of mass destruction. I need adult supervision when it comes to my mind. I need a sponsor, I need mentors, I need life coaches. I don't need to think that I am the smartest person in the room, ever. I can't cancel myself. I can't do therapy on me. No way, man! I need people. I need somebody to give me feedback. If you see something is going on with me, love me enough to tell me the truth about me and what you see. If you see me slippin', please, tell me, man!

I thank God for my life experiences with the good, the bad, and the ugly, because I personally learn more from my mistakes than my accomplishments. I am grateful that we were able to complete *Recovering From The Game*, and I'm looking froward to people reading this and getting something out of it. I hope readers say, "If this low-down bottom, carpet-cleaning, window-peeping, sleeping-outside-on-the-street addict can get clean and stay clean, I can too, one day at a time."

MY GRATITUDE

I am so excited that we are coming to the end of this project. So many people have taken the time to tell us their stories, their experiences with the lifestyles of addiction and everything that goes along with hustling in the streets. We talked to some people who you would call pimps or macs and people who were formerly boosters, but they gave up that lifestyle and they came into recovery. Their stories show that anybody can get clean if they really want to. Anybody can change. Change is not hard, it's the *resistance to change* that makes change hard. I resisted change for so long that when I finally decided to change I had to really embrace it.

I definitely want to thank all the organizations and people that I worked for or worked with when I came into recovery. From the Ozanam Center, St. Vincent DePaul, Rosemary Mcloud, Vicki, Danny and Big Fred, and all those people working at the Ozanam Center back then. All of these people helped me when I first walked in on July 18, 1995, my official clean date. Deborah Williams is the woman who opened the door for me. She wasn't even supposed to let me in because I was 86'd, but she told me, "Just lay down and don't say anything. There's a meeting tomorrow, and you're going to that meeting." Deborah gave me my last chance. Roy Washington, who we all called "Duwell," was a counselor for St. Anthony's, and I want to thank St. Vincent DePaul and St. Anthony Foundation because that's where it all started for me. It all started at 55 Jones Street. A woman named Ora did my intake, and I'm grateful for that.

I also want to thank Randy Shaw and my employer since 2013, the Tenderloin Housing Clinic, for always standing behind the vision of recovery and committing to recovery-based services. I appreciate THC's core values, all the opportunities for advancement, all the diversity from the different races, genders, and sexual orientations. I just love everybody that works for THC. I like the trailblazing that THC does. I like that, Randy Shaw, the co-founder of the Tenderloin Housing Clinic, is a rebel. Randy Shaw has that pit bull in him. When he wants to go after something, he really gets after it. and he never backs down. Some people don't agree with Randy all the time, but that's ok. I love Randy's commitment to his own belief system, and I thank him for giving me the opportunities that he has given me. He trusts me to speak my mind to the press, to voice my own personal opinions and beliefs. I get calls from San Francisco news outlets like the *Chronicle* and the *San Francisco Standard*, and from people in different leadership positions in San Francisco, all of whom were referred to talk to me by Randy Shaw. Randy knows I will say the right thing, and he knows I have love and respect for the Tenderloin Housing Clinic.

It has been a long journey to get where I am today. Going through different modalities of treatment, different philosophies, different administrations, different mayors and supervisors. But the biggest joy that I have experienced is working with the recovery population. I have been able to see somebody come into recovery, get clean and stay clean, and become productive members of society. I tell people all the time, "The only person you need to compare yourself to is the person you were before you came here." You don't need to try and compare yourself to me or anybody else. Just think about where you were. Think about your last run. Think about how you felt about what you did to your family, your loved ones, your friends. Whatever your bottom was, just think about that. Don't worry about me or the guy sitting across from you. Compare yourself to you. The old you.

I'd like to extend a special thanks to my sponsor, Roland Williams, who has been a mentor and inspiration for the past 30 years. To my Men in Motion brothers, the Staying Connected group, and my Masonic fraternity—your support has been invaluable.

I'm thankful to Mark Grey for encouraging me to create this book. It wasn't an accident that we connected, and I really appreciate you. You were the first person to put me in print with your last book, *Thank You for Sharing*. You came to interview me because people in the neighborhood told you that you had to talk to me, and that really got me thinking. It got me thinking that now is the time for me to come out with this book. Who knows how long I would have waited to come out with *Recovering From The Game* if we never met? I keep your book in my car's glove compartment because it's important to me.

I want to thank the organization Free at Last and the groups Staying Connected and Circle for Recovery. I have to mention David Lewis and Vicki Smothers, who founded Free at Last. Vicki embraced me back in the early days. There are so many heroes and sheroes out there in recovery who don't always get their flowers, but every time I see Vicki, I let her know how important she is to me. Sadly, David Lewis passed away, murdered by one of his childhood friends. I'm grateful to Dorsey Nunn, a co-founder of Free at Last who wrote *What Kind of Bird Can't Fly* and has become a good friend of mine. Dorsey started the "Ban the Box Initiative" in Washington DC and founded the nonprofit All of Us Or None (AOUON) in 2003. I have his book in my car as well.

To my beautiful wife, my Queen—thank you for being the unwavering light in my life. Your unconditional love, strength, and courage have lifted me in ways words can never fully capture. You are my rock, my inspiration, and my greatest blessing.

Thank you for always standing by my side, believing in me even in the moments I doubted myself. Your presence is a testament to grace, resilience, and the power of love. I am deeply grateful for the chapter you have written in this book, *From the Queen's Perspective*, because no story of mine would be complete without your wisdom, your truth, and your heart.

I honor you, I cherish you, and I thank you—for everything.

RECOVERY QUOTES

1. "Recovery is not for people who need it, it's for people who want it."
2. "The only journey is the one within." – Rainer Maria Rilke
3. "Fall seven times, stand up eight." – Japanese Proverb
4. "It's not the load that breaks you down, it's the way you carry it." – Lou Holtz
5. "Recovery is hard. Regret is harder."
6. "One small step today can lead to miles of success tomorrow."
7. "Strength doesn't come from what you can do. It comes from overcoming the things you thought you couldn't."
8. "You don't have to see the whole staircase, just take the first step." – Martin Luther King Jr.
9. "Progress, not perfection."
10. "Success is the sum of small efforts, repeated day in and day out." – Robert Collier
11. "The first step towards getting somewhere is to decide that you are not going to stay where you are."
12. "Rock bottom became the solid foundation on which I rebuilt my life." – J.K. Rowling
13. "Healing is an inside job."
14. "The only way out is through." – Robert Frost
15. "What lies behind us and what lies before us are tiny matters compared to what lies within us." – Ralph Waldo Emerson
16. "Addiction is the only prison where the locks are on the inside."

17. "You are stronger than you know."
18. "Believe in yourself and all that you are. Know that there is something inside you that is greater than any obstacle." – Christian D. Larson
19. "The comeback is always stronger than the setback."
20. "You don't get over an addiction by stopping using. You recover by creating a new life where it is easier not to use."
21. "Don't let the past steal your present." – Terri Guillemets
22. "It's never too late to be what you might have been." – George Eliot
23. "Recovery is an acceptance that your life is in shambles and you have to change."
24. "I am not defined by my relapses, but by my decision to remain in recovery despite them."
25. "What the caterpillar calls the end of the world, the master calls a butterfly." – Richard Bach
26. "Your best days are yet to come."
27. "Courage doesn't always roar. Sometimes courage is the quiet voice at the end of the day saying, 'I will try again tomorrow.'" – Mary Anne Radmacher
28. "You only fail when you stop trying."
29. "Courage is not having the strength to go on; it is going on when you don't have the strength." – Theodore Roosevelt
30. "Recovery didn't open the gates of heaven and let me in. Recovery opened the gates of hell and let me out."
31. "Sometimes we motivate ourselves by thinking of what we want to become. Sometimes we motivate ourselves by thinking about who we don't ever want to be again."
32. "The pain you feel today will be the strength you feel tomorrow."
33. "If you're going through hell, keep going." – Winston Churchill
34. "You may have to fight a battle more than once to win it." – Margaret Thatcher

35. "You're not going to master the rest of your life in one day. Just relax. Master the day. Then keep doing that every day."
36. "Though no one can go back and make a brand-new start, anyone can start from now and make a brand-new ending." – Carl Bard
37. "Hardships often prepare ordinary people for an extraordinary destiny." – C.S. Lewis
38. "The only person you are destined to become is the person you decide to be." – Ralph Waldo Emerson
39. "Every recovery from addiction began with one sober hour."
40. "Recovery is something that you have to work on every single day, and it's something that doesn't get a day off." – Demi Lovato
41. "It does not matter how slowly you go as long as you do not stop." – Confucius
42. "The only person you should try to be better than is the person you were yesterday."
43. "I'm not telling you it's going to be easy, I'm telling you it's going to be worth it."
44. "One of the hardest things was learning that I was worth recovery."
45. "Small steps in the right direction can turn out to be the biggest steps of your life."
46. "I can't change the direction of the wind, but I can adjust my sails to always reach my destination." – Jimmy Dean
47. "When everything seems like an uphill struggle, just think of the view from the top."
48. "Recovery is not the absence of conflict. It's the ability to handle conflict by peaceful means."
49. "You are not your past."
50. "Out of difficulties grow miracles." – Jean de La Bruyère
51. "Strength is what we gain from the madness we survive."
52. "There's no shame in beginning again, for you get a chance to build bigger and better than before."
53. "Don't quit before the miracle happens."

54. "When you can't control what's happening, challenge yourself to control how you respond to what's happening."

55. "In the midst of winter, I found there was, within me, an invincible summer." – Albert Camus

56. "One day, one moment, one breath at a time."

57. "Take pride in how far you've come. Have faith in how far you can go."

58. "It always seems impossible until it's done." – Nelson Mandela

59. "Recovery is the bridge between who you were and who you are meant to be."

60. "Let go of the life you have planned, to accept the life that is waiting for you." – Joseph Campbell

61. "We don't grow when things are easy. We grow when we face challenges."

62. "Recovery is a process. It takes time. It takes patience. It takes everything you've got."

63. "You are braver than you believe, stronger than you seem, and smarter than you think." – A.A. Milne

64. "Recovery is a journey, not a destination."

65. "If you find yourself in a hole, stop digging."

66. "Your past does not determine your future."

67. "Sobriety is not a limitation. It's a liberation."

68. "The best view comes after the hardest climb."

69. "Each day is a new beginning, and tomorrow is not yet written."

70. "Even the darkest night will end and the sun will rise." – Victor Hugo

71. "Be stronger than your strongest excuse."

72. "You didn't come this far, just to come this far."

SLANG WORDS FOR STREET DRUGS

Cannabis/Marijuana

- Weed
- Pot
- Grass
- Mary Jane
- Ganja
- Reefer
- Herb
- Dope
- Chronic
- Kush
- Bud
- Green
- Sticky icky
- Skunk
- Smoke
- Trees
- Loud
- Purple Haze
- Devil's lettuce
- Hash
- 420
- Blaze

- Sinsemilla
- Thai stick

Cocaine

- Blow
- Coke
- Snow
- Yayo
- White
- Nose candy
- Powder
- Flake
- Pearl
- Rock (for crack cocaine)
- Crack
- Base
- Hard
- Soft
- Girl
- Booger sugar
- White horse
- Sleet
- Perico

Heroin

- Smack
- H
- Junk
- Horse

- Brown sugar
- Dope
- Black tar
- China white
- Dragon
- Mud
- Skag
- Boy
- He
- Mexican brown
- Black pearl
- Black eagle
- Brown crystal
- White lady
- Thunder
- Hell dust

Methamphetamine

- Meth
- Crystal
- Crank
- Ice
- Glass
- Speed
- Tina
- Chalk
- Stove top
- Tweak
- Gak
- Go-fast
- Quartz
- Zip

- Trash
- Geeter
- Go-Go juice
- Chicken feed

Ecstasy/MDMA

- E
- Molly
- X
- Roll
- Adam
- Love drug
- Beans
- Cadillac
- Disco biscuits
- XTC
- Happy pill
- Smartees
- Scooby snacks
- Sweeties
- Candy
- Hug drug

LSD

- Acid
- Tabs
- Blotter
- Dots
- Lucy

- Window pane
- Trips
- Zen
- Cid
- Sugar cubes
- Paper acid
- Hits
- Mind candy
- Sunshine
- L
- Boomers

Psilocybin Mushrooms

- Shrooms
- Magic mushrooms
- Boomers
- Caps
- Mushies
- Cubes
- Fungus
- Golden tops
- Little smoke
- Pizza toppings
- Alice
- Blue meanies
- Sacred mushrooms
- God's flesh

Prescription Opioids (Oxycodone, Hydrocodone, etc.)

- Oxy
- Vikes

- Percs
- OC
- Hillbilly heroin
- Kickers
- Beans
- Cotton
- Roxy
- Blue heaven
- Ox
- Blue boys
- OCs
- Blues
- Killer
- 40s

Benzodiazepines (Xanax, Valium, etc.)

- Xannies
- Bars
- Benzos
- Blues
- Zannies
- Downers
- Chill pills
- Bricks
- Ladders
- Tranks
- Totem poles
- Candy bars

Ketamine

- Special K

- K
- Cat tranquilizer
- Vitamin K
- Jet
- Kit-Kat
- Super acid
- Green
- Honey oil
- Horse trank
- Kay

Fentanyl

- Fenty
- Dance Fever
- Apache
- China girl
- Murder 8
- TNT
- Great bear
- Jackpot

Other Drugs and Slang

- **Lean (Codeine with soda)**
  - Sizzurp
  - Purple drank
  - Dirty Sprite
  - Barre
  - Syrup
  - Texas tea
  - Drank

○ Tsikuni
- **Bath Salts (Synthetic cathinones)**
  ○ Cloud 9
  ○ Lunar wave
  ○ Vanilla sky
  ○ Scarface
  ○ Bloom
  ○ White lightning
  ○ Plant fertilizer
- **Spice/K2 (Synthetic cannabinoids)**
  ○ Fake weed
  ○ Black Mamba
  ○ Genie
  ○ Scooby Snax
  ○ Moon rocks
  ○ K2
  ○ Zohai
  ○ Red X dawn
  ○ Bliss
  ○ Blueberry Haze
- **PCP (Phencyclidine)**
  ○ Angel dust
  ○ Wet
  ○ Sherm
  ○ Boat
  ○ Hog
  ○ Wack
  ○ Embalming fluid
  ○ Ozone
  ○ Rocket fuel
  ○ Love boat
- **Inhalants**
  ○ Whippets

- Poppers
- Rush
- Snappers
- Glue
- Huff
- Air blast
- Balloons
- Locker room

- **GHB (Gamma-Hydroxybutyrate)**
  - G
  - Liquid ecstasy
  - Georgia homeboy
  - G-juice
  - Soap
  - Gook
  - Scoop
  - Cherry meth

- **DMT (Dimethyltryptamine)**
  - Dimitri
  - The spirit molecule
  - Businessman's trip
  - Fantasia
  - 45-minute psychosis

- **Salvia**
  - Magic mint
  - Sally-D
  - Maria pastora
  - Diviner's sage

RICHARD BEAL

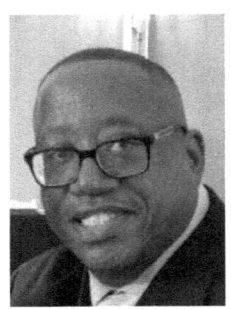

Richard currently lives in Antioch, but his heart is always in the streets of San Francisco. Known in the Tenderloin as the "TL Ambassador for Recovery," he has been working in the city for the last twenty-seven years. Richard came to San Francisco in 1985, and lived there struggling with his addiction and homelessness for the next ten years. During his addiction, he was arrested numerous times, first in Richmond, CA, then in Oakland, CA, and he finally landed at San Francisco County Jail. On July 18, 1995, Richard entered Ozanam Detox on 8th & Howard Streets. On July 20, 1995, he entered St. Anthony's Foundation Rehabilitation Program's Seton Hall in San Francisco, and he has been in recovery ever since.

Today Richard is the Director of Transitional Housing for Tenderloin Housing Clinic. He instituted an annual Recovery Day in Boedekker Park in 2021. Richard is the chairperson of the Direct Action Committee of the San Francisco Reentry Council, and he is an Advanced Certified Relapse Prevention Counselor under CENAPS Corporation. Richard is a sponsor, mentor, life coach, and loving, caring child of God.

MARK GREY

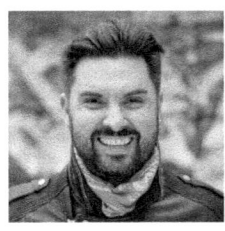

Mark resides in San Francisco. His work focuses on topics such as addiction, mental illness, dual diagnosis, teen homelessness, recovery, and other current events such as the covid-19 pandemic and its effects on society as a whole. Today, armed with a wealth of knowledge due to personal experiences with these topics, Mark hopes to help those caught in the grips of the madness that is addiction. As of 2025, Mark has published nine books and is always working on new and exciting book projects.

www.ingramcontent.com/pod-product-compliance
Lightning Source LLC
Chambersburg PA
CBHW061748120626
46550CB00005B/1927

* 9 7 9 8 9 9 2 9 0 5 6 0 1 *